# Reverence in Healing

# Reverence in Healing

## Honoring Strengths without Trivializing Suffering

Edited by David A. Crenshaw

JASON ARONSON
*Lanham • Boulder • New York • Toronto • Plymouth, UK*

Published by Jason Aronson
An imprint of Rowman & Littlefield Publishers, Inc.
A wholly owned subsidiary of The Rowman & Littlefield Publishing Group, Inc.
4501 Forbes Boulevard, Suite 200, Lanham, Maryland 20706
http://www.rowmanlittlefield.com

Estover Road, Plymouth PL6 7PY, United Kingdom



British Library Cataloguing in Publication Information Available

**Library of Congress Cataloging-in-Publication Data**

Reverence in healing : honoring strengths without trivializing suffering / edited by David A. Crenshaw.
p. cm.
Includes bibliographical references and index.
ISBN 978-0-7657-0658-4 (cloth : alk. paper) — ISBN 978-0-7657-0660-7 (electronic)
1. Healing—Psychological aspects. 2. Respect. 3. Medical care. I. Crenshaw, David A.
R726.5.R48 2010
615.5—dc22 2009030442

∞™ The paper used in this publication meets the minimum requirements of American National Standard for Information Sciences—Permanence of Paper for Printed Library Materials, ANSI/NISO Z39.48-1992.

Printed in the United States of America

Dedicated to Robert Brooks, a true pioneer in strengths-based healing

# Contents

# Acknowledgments

This book is dedicated to Robert Brooks, a faculty member of Harvard Medical School. After reading his writings in collaboration with his good friend, Sam Goldstein, Ph.D., on the themes of resilience, self-esteem, motivation, and family relationships I was eager to hear him speak. I was told by numerous people that he was one of the most dynamic, engaging, and charismatic speakers in our field. I finally had my chance when Robert Brooks was invited to deliver a keynote speech on the occasion of the Astor Home for Children's 50th Anniversary Conference. Although I had high expectations, I was completely unprepared for what I experienced as the most dynamic and effective speaker I've ever heard in any field. I laughed so hard I am afraid I may have made a spectacle of myself but his humorous way of delivering his serious and important message added immeasurably to the impact. Robert Brooks's storytelling was spellbinding; his delivery was marked by his masterful use of timing; and his effective use of pauses and changes in affect to punctuate key points left me filled with awe and admiration. We are so fortunate in our field to have such a dynamic and effective messenger delivering such an important message. Robert Brooks challenges us to go beyond the pathology mind-set that has dominated the field from Freud to this very day. This mind-set is based on the medical model and fits well when a pathologist examines a specimen in the laboratory; it is very limiting when trying to understand the rich complexity of a human being. Robert Brooks, who contributes a cornerstone chapter in this book, and Edith Lawrence, who also with a colleague writes a chapter in this book, are pioneers in developing the strengths-based mind-set. Edith Lawrence applies the strengths-based approach to work with families, resulting in a book with David Waters in 1993, *Competence, Courage, and Change: An*

*Approach to Family Therapy*. Robert Brooks in the early 1970s at McLean Hospital and in his private practice began using a strengths-based approach in therapy and developed his Creative Characters Storytelling Technique. He taught the resilience/strengths-based approach in lectures and writing and expanded this model in collaboration with Sam Goldstein in the late 1990s to nurturing and parenting resilient children, culminating in their book *Raising Resilient Children* in 2001. In recent years Robert Brooks has consulted with numerous schools and has lectured widely on highlighting and building on strengths of children in schools, and even developing this empowering approach to people within the workplace. As a result, he is frequently sought as a consultant to corporations.

Considered to be one of the top and most highly sought speakers today and a leading authority on resilience in children, adolescents, and adults, he is also a person I've come to respect and admire for his reverence in all the inspiring work he does. When you focus as much on what is right with people as you do on what is wrong with them, you are showing reverence. He is a passionate, committed, deeply caring, and genuine man. I am proud to dedicate this book to him as a kindred spirit, valued friend, and a towering, inspiring figure that touches the hearts of all who are fortunate to come to know him.

# I

# INTRODUCTION AND OVERVIEW OF REVERENCE IN HEALING

# 1

# Reverence in the Healing Process

*David A. Crenshaw*

> Those who have the humility of a child may find again the key to reverence for, and kinship with, all life.
>
> —J. Allen Boone

Reverence is exemplified in a sense of awe, a profound respect for all living things but especially evident in our attitude toward the most vulnerable among us, particularly children but even animals, plants, and trees. The contemporary philosopher Paul Woodruff (2001) explained that reverence was a highly cherished virtue in the ancient cultures of China and Greece but seems to have been forgotten in modern Western culture. Woodruff explained that although reverence is hard to define, when it is missing in culture, history reveals that things tend to fall apart. Woodruff (2001) stated, "Reverence begins in a deep understanding of human limitations; from this grows the capacity to be in awe of whatever we believe lies outside our control—God, truth, justice, nature, even death. The capacity for awe, as it grows, brings with it the capacity for respecting fellow human beings, flaws and all. This in turn fosters the ability to be ashamed when we show moral flaws exceeding the normal human allotment. The Greeks before Plato saw reverence as one of the bulwarks of society, and the immediate followers of Confucius in China thought much the same" (pp. 3–4). Reverence is especially reflected in our attitudes toward children. Woodruff explained, "To forget that you are only human, to think that you can act like a god—that is the opposite of reverence. Ancient Greeks thought that tyranny was the height of irreverence, and they gave the famous name *hubris* to the crimes of tyrants. An irreverent soul is arrogant and shameless, unable to feel awe in the face of things higher than itself.

As a result, an irreverent soul is unable to feel respect for people it sees as lower than itself—ordinary people, prisoners, children" (p. 4). Woodruff added, "And any of us is better for remembering that there is someone, or Someone, to whom we are children; in this frame of mind we are more likely to treat all children with respect" (p. 4). Thus the true measure of reverence is not how we treat our superiors or our colleagues but how we respond to those more vulnerable among us. I would never refer a patient to a psychiatrist who treated his or her secretary badly.

In work with children or adults nothing is more fundamental or crucial to success than an attitude of reverence. It is one of the building blocks of the therapeutic alliance that empirically has been demonstrated to play a crucial role in healing both with children and adults (Kazdin, 2005). In healing work with children one of the ways we show reverence is to notice the pain that they can't tell us about in words but reveal in their eyes or by words not spoken.

### Look Deeply into the Eyes of a Child

Look deeply into the eyes of a child.
Children hide their pain in all kinds of ways.
But they can't hide it in their eyes.
Look deeply into the eyes of a child.
Do you see even a glimmer of light?
Light reveals that the divine spark within the soul is still present.
Look deeply in the eyes of a child.
Darkness reveals the child's eyes saw what no child should ever see.
And never wants to see again.
Look deeply in the eyes of a child.
Although you may see only darkness, don't despair.
Light can once again enter to rekindle the spirit of a child.
Look deeply in the eyes of a child.
Know that even in the darkest corner of the child's eyes, there may be a glimmer of light; a tiny glow to let you know that the divine spark is not easily extinguished.

—David A. Crenshaw

### Silence Is Not Golden

Cicero said, "Their very silence is a loud cry."
Silence is a poignant presence by virtue of absence, the absence of spoken words.
Silence speaks volumes, when a child is silenced.
What is not said is far more important than any words spoken.
The spaces and pauses between the words spoken may like a secret code, in the language of silence reveal the untold stories that words can't tell.
Silence in children who were silenced is not golden.
Listen carefully to the language of silence, the words unspoken; the stories untold.

Only if we hear what is unsaid will children find their voice to tell us their stories in words.

—David A. Crenshaw

## REVERENCE IN HEALING

In psychotherapy, the healing process can't begin in earnest without reverence for the people we would heal. Reverence is rarely talked about in the mental health disciplines but, as Woodruff (2001) noted to be true in the wider culture, without reverence "things tend to fall apart." James Garbarino (1999) used the term "divine spark" to describe that special essence that babies arrive with on birth. There is a "specialness" with the newborn; an innocence that can't easily be defined but strongly sensed by anyone who fixes a gaze on the infant. This specialness, the "divine spark" becomes more indistinct as infants grow and develop but it still exists if we are able to look past the various behavioral and emotional masks put on by children to protect against vulnerability. Reverence, awe, profound respect for the specialness of a child can facilitate growth and healing whether in psychotherapy, parenting, or teaching. Children can tell when they are viewed with reverence; they can also tell when they are not.

## THE CONCEPT OF REVERENCE IN PSYCHOTHERAPY

In spite of the crucial importance of reverence to healing of children and adults there is little mention of reverence in the psychological literature. Ira Byock (2007), working in the Palliative Medicine Department at Dartmouth Hitchcock Medical Center, discussed reverence in the context of people confronting death. Reverence for life and for other human beings comes most sharply into focus when we are forced to realize how precious the gift of life is and also how fleeting and fragile it is. Byock stated, "The confrontation with death lays bare the spiritual core of the human condition. Human spirituality arises in response to the awe-inspiring and terrifying mystery of life and the universe. We reflexively seek to make meaning of our experience in the world and make or strengthen our connections to others" (p. 436).

Depth psychology has traditionally showed a deep reverence for the soul, its search for meaning, purpose, and meaningful connection with others. Depth psychology and therapy recognize that in nearly every human being there is a longing for a spiritual dimension that may or may not include a religious affiliation that is seeking inspiration, to be deeply moved, capable of awe and reverence, even among those who don't believe in God (Culliford, 2002). Likewise in a depth psychology framework, E. Mark Stern (1966) discussed the "instrumental" and "sacramental" approaches to experience in psychotherapy (see chapter 4 in this book for Stern's most recent thinking on reverence in psychotherapy). The instrumental approach considers the patient's past as something to overcome through emotional insight and regards the present as a problem to be resolved through adjustment to reality, an approach which treats the therapeutic situation as something apart from the patient's life. The sacramental approach treats the past as worthy of respect and the present as an experience which can be transformed through concerned and appreciative confrontation, an approach which seeks to integrate the treatment experience into the patient's life. The sacramental approach, in short, expresses reverence for the patient and his or her emotional experiences. Stern, in discussing reverence for the experiences of the patient in therapy, stated, "The personal encounter which leads to a real relationship between persons is of peculiar significance in the therapeutic situation. Classically, the therapist is present in a fashion somewhat divorced from what is generally known as human presence. His unperturbed surface allows the patient to create and live out other relationships in great variety; the therapist may be anybody to the patient, anybody except the self he is outside the therapeutic hour. The therapist who reveres experience does not thus stand apart. He *accompanies* (italics in the original text) his patient to fulfillment" (1966, p. 281). The fact that it was necessary to go back more than forty years to Stern's article to locate even the mention of the word reverence in relation to the psychotherapy process is consistent with Woodruff's (2001) thesis that reverence is a forgotten virtue not only in modern culture but also in psychotherapy.

John O'Donohue (2004), the late Irish poet and philosopher, like Woodruff also lamented the loss of reverence in contemporary culture. O'Donohue explained, "Our culture has little respect for privacy; we no longer recognize the sacred zone around each person. We feel we have a right to blunder unannounced into any area we wish. Because we have lost reverence of approach, we should not be too surprised at the lack of quality and beauty in our experience. At the heart of things is a secret law of balance and when our approach is respectful, sensitive and worthy, gifts of healing, challenge and creativity open to us. A gracious approach is the key that unlocks the treasure of encounter" (p. 24). While O'Donohue was not focusing on psychotherapy, his concept of a reverent, respectful, sensitive, worthy, and gracious approach is ripe with implications for how we engage in the healing process. Without reverence, our inquiries may be experienced by our child or adult patients as intrusive, insensitive, and disrespectful. Instead of creating an invitation to openness and disclosure we may instead foment protective defensiveness and closure in people.

## RESILIENCE, COMPETENCE, AND STRENGTHS-BASED APPROACHES

One of the "lone voices in the wilderness" has been Robert Brooks (1993; Brooks & Goldstein, 2004) who has strongly advocated for a resilience and strengths-based approach to parenting, educating, and healing our youth. Brooks in chapter 2 of this book gives a comprehensive overview of the power of "mind-sets" and his personal journey to honor and celebrate dignity, hope, and resilience in children. This book is dedicated to him for his groundbreaking work in challenging the prevailing pathology mind-set approach, which derives from the medical model that examines disease under the lab microscope and through the high technology imaging techniques available today. It is a limiting model for understanding and healing a person. Because it overlooks what is "right" within the person it lacks reverence.

David Waters and Edith Lawrence (1993) also significantly contributed to this shift in the "pathology mind-set" in work with families by emphasizing competence, courage, love, hope, and vision in families. Waters and Lawrence didn't ignore pathology but rather found the seeds of strength within the family often embedded in their pathology. This refreshing approach to work with families brought into the therapy room a focus not just on dysfunction and illness, but health and competence, strength, and important qualities rarely talked about before in family therapy including the family's vision, hope, and their love and compassion (see chapter 10 for Edith Lawrence's and Amanda Sovik-Johnston's detailed discussion of the competency approach in family therapy).

## MULTIPLE DIMENSIONS OF REVERENCE

### Reverence for the Person

In addition to the reverence, sensitivity, and profound respect for the suffering of a person, reverence is also needed for the strengths, talents, positive personal qualities, courage, hope, and vision of people as well as their capacities for empathy, generosity, love, and compassion. Antwone Fisher (2001) wrote a book about his life that was made into a deeply moving film about his harsh experiences in the foster care system. Fisher has distinguished himself as an author, poet, teacher, and screenwriter in Hollywood. Antwone Fisher is far more than a person who suffered abuse as a child. His strength, courage, and determination have inspired countless people to believe that even the harshest beginnings in life are possible to overcome.

## Reverence for Families

Families in mental health treatment in the past often felt stigmatized, sometimes blamed, or, even worse, on occasion demonized as a result of the psychiatric suffering of one or more family members. While it is true that a small percentage of families are destructive and inflict suffering on their children, the vast majority of parents and extended families do the best they can to raise and support their children. They are too often blamed, made to feel guilty, and rarely receive proper credit for the ways they nurture, support, and guide their children day in and day out. I often marvel at the heroic efforts made by single parent families, mothers or fathers, to meet the needs of their children in the face of overwhelming demands. It is so easy to blame parents when something goes wrong. These parents like the children deserve to be treated with reverence.

## Reverence for Humanity

Global reverence has been noted as essential for cross-cultural understanding. Maraj Desai (2007) discussed the necessary ingredients for cross-cultural understanding "that not only has taken place, but also lies ahead of us when one is able to listen to and respectfully dwell with the other, slowly and in a manner of shy reverence" (p. 313). In a cross-cultural study comparing reverence for mothers in Ecuadorian and Euro-American cultures, it was found among college students that Ecuadorians display higher levels of mother reverence than Euro-Americans (Mealy, Stephan, & Abalakina-Paap, 2006). These findings are consistent with the contention of Woodruff (2001) that reverence is particularly a declining value in American culture.

Ralph Ellis (2004) in his book, *Love and the Abyss: An Essay on Finitude and Value,* suggested that in a modern world where so many feel dispensable, the value of humanity needs to be reclaimed. He argued that meaning in this world comes in relation to our fellow humans and that human life is to be celebrated and appreciated. It is simply human life per se that we ought to regard with awe-filled reverence.

## Reverence for our Environment

Conservationists advocate reverence for our earth and its resources (Low, 2007). The survival of our planet depends on changing our wasteful, irreverent ways particularly in the United States. A place of healing called "Forget Me Not Farm" is a nationally acclaimed and award-winning animal-assisted and horticultural therapy program located in Santa Rosa, California (Rossiter, 2006), that stresses reverence for all living things. It has been in operation since 1992 and works collaboratively with community resources to provide healing, bonding, and attachment experiences for at-risk children. Children learn how to take care of animals including bathing, grooming, and feeding the resident farm animals. Likewise, they learn about the natural life cycle by planting seeds and tending plants in the organic garden. Learning to tenderly care for animals and plants provides an emotionally healing experience and among the values learned are compassion, empathy, gentleness, accountability for one's actions, respect for self and others, and reverence for all living things.

O'Donohue (2004) discussed how we lack appreciation in the modern world for the beauty that surrounds us in nature. Reverence for beauty and respect for the fragile nature of all living things as well as our natural environment are essential if we are going to preserve the planet for future generations. Reverence for the beauty of our world enhances all of us. O'Donohue stated, "To behold beauty dignifies your life; it heals you and calls you out beyond the smallness of your own self-limitation to experience new horizons. To experience beauty is to have your life enlarged" (p. 20). There is also beauty in every person. But like the beauty of the natural world we don't always notice, both the beauty within ourselves and in others. Reverence for beauty in the world around us and in a person requires that we become more conscious and open to its gracious invitations on a daily basis.

Beauty: Do We Notice?

Beauty within us
Beauty around us
Beauty that elevates the spirit
Beauty that nourishes the soul
Beauty in simple acts of kindness
Beauty in forgiveness
Beauty in acceptance
Beauty in compassion
Beauty in love
Beauty in loyalty
Do we notice?

Beauty in animals
Beauty in nature
Beauty in flowers
Beauty in smiles
Beauty in holding on
Beauty in letting go
Beauty in a life well-lived
Beauty in courage facing suffering
Beauty in dying with dignity
Beauty in reverence
Do we notice?

Beauty in respect
Beauty in sensitivity
Beauty in humility
Beauty in strength
Beauty in children and adults playing
Beauty in laughter
Beauty in remembering
Beauty in forgetting
Beauty in sharing
Beauty in caring
Do we notice?

Beauty in helping
Beauty in giving
Beauty in gracious receiving
Beauty in consoling a child
Beauty in friendship
Beauty in family ties
Beauty in intimacy
Beauty in trust
Beauty in the heart
Beauty in the soul
Do we notice?

Beauty in tenderness
Beauty in hugs
Beauty in touch
Beauty in reconciliation
Beauty in dedication
Beauty in passion
Beauty in reflection
Do we notice?

—David A. Crenshaw

## THE PATHOLOGY MIND-SET

Mental health field professionals in all disciplines are trained to identify, classify, and treat all forms of pathology. The Diagnostic Statistical Manual is the "bible" for mental health professionals for classification of various symptoms and disorders. The "bible" makes little or no mention of strengths, competencies, talents, or redeeming qualities. This is a limiting, demeaning way of viewing people. The various diagnostic codes don't begin to capture the rich complexity of the human beings we seek to help, and no consideration is given to what is right with them, only what is wrong with them. In approaching people this way we do not show reverence. People are far more than any diagnostic code can adequately delineate.

A more subtle way of showing lack of reverence in the mental health field is the descriptive language we use to describe various forms of psychopathology. Jerome Kagan (1998), in a lecture entitled "How We Become Who We Are" at the Family Therapy Networker Symposium, explained that we should never use language like the "aggressive child" or "the fearful child" or the "phobic child." He observed that no child is aggressive, fearful, or phobic all the time. These terms have no value unless we specify under what conditions and in what context these behaviors occur. The use of such terms that is quite prevalent in the field (I acknowledge that I am remiss as well) can leave a child or the family feeling that this is a fixed attribute of their personhood. When we use such pathologizing language, we lack reverence.

## LACK OF REVERENCE AND "SPIRIT BREAKING"

Those who seek to heal are entrusted with a special responsibility to avoid harm. Patricia Deegan (1990) noted that when human services workers do not show reverence toward the recipients of their services the spirit of the person may be broken. When the dignity of the person, whether child or adult, is not respected or even worse assaulted, it results in a rupture in relatedness that can cause injury to the spirit of a person. While there are many wonderful, compassionate mental health professions, as in any profession there are those who do not show reverence for those who seek their help.

The same is true in education. While the vast majority of teachers are dedicated to their students and play an immensely valuable role in society by educating each new generation of children, there are a few who cause great harm by their lack of reverence for children. Those teachers would be surprised to know that an adult in a therapist's office sometimes still remembers vividly the humiliation suffered during kindergarten or first grade with such a teacher—their spirit was broken in a way that still seeks repair years later. The same lack of reverence can be shown by parents, physicians, teachers, or anyone in human services with the same unfortunate results. When human services are delivered in a dehumanizing or demeaning manner, we risk breaking the spirit of the child, adult, or family. I fear that the overemphasis on a pathology-based classification system can result in a dehumanizing experience for consumers accessing mental health services. We are reminded again that without reverence things tend to fall apart.

## REVERENCE FOR SUFFERING

In prior books written for mental health professionals, I attempted to focus on strengths, but like my colleagues, I focused far more on the woundedness and suffering of children and adults (Crenshaw, 2006, 2008a, 2008b). The suffering and wounds of children and adults need to be treated with reverence, with respect, and sensitivity. Evidence that sharing emotional pain is beneficial comes from studies that disclosure of traumatic experiences improves the immune system (Kemeny & Schedlowski, 2007) and that disclosure of traumatic experiences even significantly reduced the healing time of surgical wounds as compared to a control group who did not disclose emotionally painful experiences prior to the surgical procedure (Weinman, Ebrecht, Scott, Walburn, & Dyson, 2008).

Injuries to the Spirit

Hegel said, "The wounds of the spirit heal and leave no scars behind."
The great philosopher was, of course, correct.
Even the high tech imaging techniques of medical science do not show visible wounds to the spirit
But do not be misled.
Of all injuries children suffer, none are as devastating as the crushing of their spirit.

—David A. Crenshaw

We should never trivialize or minimize the suffering of another. But nor should we focus exclusively on the suffering and miss everything else that is important in defining the person. When we overfocus on deficits, whether in parenting, teaching, or in therapy, we are showing a lack of reverence. Such lack of appreciation for the richness and complexity of people leaves them feeling stuck and helpless. If we assume damage, we will always find it. If we expect trauma our expectation will be confirmed. If we can only think and evaluate from a pathology mind-set we will miss the true essence of the person who has turned to us for help and understanding.

## DEHUMANIZING CULTURAL INFLUENCES

Mental health care is not the only place where reverence for the person is essential and too often lacking, as Woodruff (2001) observed it seems to be a forgotten virtue in contemporary life.

### Dehumanizing Practices in the Health Care System

A common complaint in the health care system by both physicians and patients is that the volume of patients that physicians need to see to maintain their incomes, particularly if they take insurance, interferes with the physician being able to spend adequate time with patients, to really listen to and understand their concerns and answer their questions. Many physicians are just as frustrated as their patients in this regard because they entered medicine in order to practice the healing arts and they value their relationships with patients.

A startling example of how dehumanizing our current health care system has become, was my experience of discovering one night in the parking lot outside of my office a man on a bitter cold winter night lying on his back. He was trembling, cold, and was experiencing chest pains and weakness in arms and limbs. I put blankets on him and called 911 while he begged me not to call because he said he didn't have health insurance and couldn't pay for the ambulance or the hospital. The experience shook me to the core. When the ambulance loaded him up and headed for the nearest hospital, I felt a deep sense of shame. How could such a dehumanizing system develop in the most advanced country in the modern world?

## Dehumanizing Practices in Education

In the hypercompetitive modern world, legislative and regulatory mandates, although well-intended to make American students more able to compete for jobs in the competitive global economy, has unwittingly created pressure for teachers to teach to a test and perhaps not see the child but rather a set of test scores. While the vast majority of teachers are committed to the well-being and growth of their students, these pressures are felt by students and teachers alike in every school in the country. For some students and teachers these higher demands and expectations work well but there are a significant number of students who are disenfranchised due to these higher standards that they can't meet. Likewise, the pressure on teachers to prepare students for the state mandated tests do not permit them to provide the help and support that some students require to keep up with the more intense pace. In addition, due to fiscal constraints impacting school budgets, sports, drama, music, and the arts, along with vocational technology opportunities are increasingly vulnerable to cuts. Those students who are unable to experience success in strictly academic pursuits are deprived of these alternative ways to be validated for their talents and capabilities.

## Dehumanizing Practices in the Workplace

Major corporations in order to compete in the global marketplace strive for a high-performance culture in the workplace. In some corporations, employees in various divisions compete with each other, with those ranked at the bottom facing the risk of losing their jobs even if everyone on the team is achieving at a superior level. This creates an extremely unhealthy workplace environment with employees experiencing a steady state of threat even if they are keeping up with the pace. An employee, for example, may feel compelled to work online at midnight if the manager of the workgroup is online sending e-mails that are being responded to by other members of the team. Employees feel they are dispensable and disposable, and this is a glaring example of lack of reverence in the workplace. The lack of reverence to our collective detriment is seen in multiple domains in our culture, in health care, in education, and in the workplace.

## HONORING RESILIENCE WITHOUT MINIMIZING SUFFERING: THE DELICATE BALANCE

A strengths-based approach that honors resilience in people is one that is respectful and reverent. A reverent, strengths-based approach is more a mind-set than a particular method of therapy. Reverence and the appreciation of the strengths of a child, adult, or family can be integral to virtually any theoretical orientation or therapeutic method.

The art of healing requires reverence for the delicate balances that are inherent in psychotherapy. While the thesis of this book is that there has been an imbalance in the mental health field that needs to be corrected due to an overemphasis on pathology to the exclusion of a focus on resilience and appreciation of strengths, clinical sensitivity is needed to avoid an overcorrection. When a child, an adult, or a family heroically battle to overcome formidable odds, we should celebrate their courage, their strength, their determination, and resilience. It is remarkable what some people are able to survive and their stories inspire and strengthen us all. We risk, however, in our celebration of strengths and resilience unwittingly conveying the message that we don't honor or respect suffering or sacrifices people made along the way. Unintentionally, we may be so focused on their accomplishments that they are left with the feeling that we are trivializing what they have survived. Even worse is the erroneous expectation that everyone can be heroic and resilient, if they just have enough willpower. Not everyone can be resilient. Sometime the circumstances of a person's life are so toxic that it overwhelms even the best of coping resources, and resilience. It was discovered during World War II that 60 straight days of frontline combat was the maximum that could be endured without psychiatric breakdown regardless of how strong the soldier. There is a limit of human endurance. It is important to show reverence for those human limits and the suffering that people endure even when they are able to heroically surmount extreme hardship and adversity in life. In treatment this is a delicate balance that healers need to achieve with sensitivity, respect, and reverence for the person, that includes appreciation of both their strengths and their suffering.

Another related delicate balance that requires great sensitivity and reverence in the healing process is the therapeutic task of facilitating hope. Jerome Frank, one of the earlier pioneers in the study of psychotherapy, identified creating hope and combating demoralization as one of the salient goals of psychotherapy. Psychotherapists of all stripes adopt this as a central tenet of their work and rightly so. But even the creation of hope requires sensitivity to a delicate balance. Hope is what keeps a person going when facing a debilitating illness or combat in the military, or occupational or business setbacks. Hope is essential to psychological coping and survival. As the late psychoanalyst Walter Bonime taught me, hope is also potentially dangerous. If people are in a daily struggle against formidable odds, their survival may depend on keeping their expectations low. Kenneth Hardy and Tracy Laszloffy (2005) called this the "survival orientation" and James Garbarino (1999) called it "terminal thinking." If your hopes and dreams are repeatedly crushed, you will not dare let your hopes get too high because if you are disappointed again that setback may prove to be one too many; it may simply be more than you can bear.

Still another challenge for the would-be healer is showing reverence for the suffering of the child, adult, or family without being engulfed and overwhelmed with the pain. This too is a delicate balance. One of the occupational hazards of healers is compassion fatigue (Figley, 2002). If therapists are too identified with the pain of the sufferer when carried to an absurd length, the sufferer may feel compelled to comfort the healer. In those cases the unresolved pain of the healer becomes activated by the pain of the sufferer resulting in a load that overwhelms the healer. Healers must take responsibility for care of their selves (Crenshaw, 2008a). This too is a delicate balance. In order for healers to extend themselves in ways that are reverential, they must also show reverence for self. Healers need to monitor their case loads, to make sure they keep a balance between cases that require intensive care and those that require the standard level of care. Healers must monitor the balance between their investment in their professional life and attention to family, friends, and care of self including adequate exercise, recreation, relaxation, playfulness, nutrition, and rest. Healers will eventually hit a wall if they don't maintain a balance between compassionate giving in their professional lives and giving in relationships and activities in their personal lives that nurture and replenish them.

This book is about reverence in healing with a group of outstanding contributors discussing strengths-based and resilience-based approaches in various treatment settings and weaved into a variety of treatment methods ranging from interventions in Head Start, play therapy, child and adolescent therapy with separate chapters on teen girls and boys, strengths-based assessment and healing of families, including military families and culturally diverse families. In addition, strengths-based approaches are described in foster care, in juvenile detention, in community-based programs, in group homes serving at-risk children and in treatment of trauma. James Garbarino of Loyola University in chapter 3 writes about the role of spirituality in healing and the need for reverence for this important dimension in the lives of many people. Each of the chapters expand on the advantages of a strengths-based reverent approach to healing within their specific setting or working with their specific clinical population as compared to the more typical and less reverent pathology mind-set. This book does not maintain that pathology can be simply ignored or overlooked but a sensitive and reverent balance must be achieved by honoring both the suffering and resilience of people. Reverence to a large extent depends on where you put the punctuation!

## REFERENCES

Brooks, R. (1993). *The search for islands of competence.* Presentation at the Fifth Annual Conference of CHADD (Children and Adults with Attention Deficit / Hyperactivity Disorder). San Diego, CA.

Brooks, R., & Goldstein, S. (2004). *The power of resilience: Achieving balance, confidence, and personal strength in your life.* New York: McGraw-Hill.

Byock, I. R. (2007). To life! Reflections on spirituality, palliative practice, and politics. *American Journal of Hospice & Palliative Medicine, 23*(6), 436–438.

Crenshaw, D. A. (2006). *Evocative strategies in child and adolescent psychotherapy.* Lanham, MD: Jason Aronson.

Crenshaw, D. A. (Ed.). (2008a). *Child and adolescent psychotherapy: Wounded spirits and healing paths.* Lanham, MD: Lexington Books.

Crenshaw, D. A. (2008b). *Therapeutic engagement of children and adolescents.* Lanham, MD: Jason Aronson.

Culliford, L. (2002). Spirituality and clinical care. *British Medical Journal, 325* (7378), 1434–1435.

Deegan, P. E. (1990). Spirit breaking: When the helping professions hurt. *The Humanistic Psychologist, 18*(3), 301–313.

Desai, M. U. (2007). Review of Heidegger, Rorty, and the Eastern thinkers: A hermeneutics of cross-cultural understanding. *Journal of Phenomenological Psychology, 38*(2), 313–316.

Ellis, R. D. (2004). *Love and the abyss: An essay on finitude and value.* Chicago: Open Court Publishing Company.

Figley, C. (2002). *Treating compassion fatigue.* New York: Psychology Press.

Fisher, A. Q. (2001). *Finding fish: A memoir.* New York: William Morrow.

Garbarino, J. (1999). *Lost boys: Why our sons turn violent and how we can save them.* New York: Anchor Books.

Hardy, K. V., & Laszloffy, T. (2005). *Teens who hurt: Clinical interventions to break the cycle of adolescent violence.* New York: Guilford Press.

Kagan, J. (1998). *How we become who we are.* Presentation at the Family Therapy Networker Symposium. Washington, DC.

Kazdin, A. E. (2005). Treatment outcomes, common factors, and continued neglect of mechanisms of change. *Clinical Psychology: Science and Practice, 12*, 184–188.

Kemeny, M., & Schedlowski, M. (2007). Understanding the interaction between psychosocial stress and immune-related diseases: A stepwise progression. *Brain, Behavior, and Immunity, 21*(8), 1009–1018.

Low, B. S. (2007). Behavioral ecology of conservation in traditional societies. In D. J. Penn & I. Mysterud (Eds.), *Evolutionary perspectives on environmental problems* (pp. 67–79). New Brunswick, NJ: Transaction Publishers.

Mealy, M., Stephan, W. G., & Abalakina-Paap, M. (2006). Reverence for mothers in Ecuadorian and Euro-American culture. *Journal of Cross-Cultural Psychology, 37*(4), 465–484.

O'Donohue, J. (2004). *Beauty: The invisible embrace.* New York: HarperCollins.

Rossiter, S. (2006). A healing place: Forget Me Not Farm. *Annals of the American Psychotherapy Association, 9*(1), 30–32.

Stern, E. M. (1966). Psychotherapy: Reverence for experience. *Journal of Existentialism, 6*(23), 279–287.

Waters, D., & Lawrence, E. (1993). *Competence, courage & change: An approach to family therapy.* New York: Norton.

Weinman, J., Ebrecht, M., Scott, S., Walburn, J., & Dyson, M. (2008). Enhanced wound healing after emotional disclosure intervention. *British Journal of Health Psychology, 13*, 95–102.

Woodruff, P. (2001). *Reverence: Renewing a forgotten virtue.* New York: Oxford University Press.

# 2

# Power of Mind-Sets: A Personal Journey to Nurture Dignity, Hope, and Resilience in Children

*Robert Brooks*

I am honored that David Crenshaw has dedicated this book to me and that he invited me to contribute a chapter. David is a person whom I greatly admire both as a warm and caring man and a gifted therapist. He possesses great empathy and compassion, enabling him to enter the world of children and gain their trust, heal their emotional wounds, and nurture their hope and resilience. He is a kindred spirit, an individual who appreciates that while we must never neglect to address the problems that burden children, we can do so most effectively by identifying and reinforcing their strengths.

## THE BEGINNING OF MY JOURNEY

In reflecting upon the message I wish to convey in this chapter, my thoughts drift back more than 40 years to the beginning of my career as a clinical psychologist and to the rich journey I have experienced since that time. Psychology was my third major in college and I was pleased that as a senior I finally discovered a subject that triggered my interest and passion. I entered graduate school eager to become a psychologist and therapist and to help others.

I found my initial experiences as a therapist disconcerting. I was plagued by doubts and questions, wondering, "What is therapy? What are the goals of therapy? What impact can I have on the lives of others? What impact do I want to have?" Like many novices, I struggled to make sense of my role as a clinician. Unfortunately, a convergence of my uncertainty and the state of the mental health field at that time contributed to an atmosphere in which

I and many other therapists too quickly cast blame on patients for a lack of progress in treatment.

Blame crept into my interpretation of what was transpiring in therapy. When my patients of any age did not improve, I questioned their motivation to change. If my best efforts to nurture a relationship with them did not lead to a feeling of connectedness, I wondered how much they wanted to work with me and confront their problems. In describing my patients, my therapy process notes were filled with words such as "resistant" or "oppositional" or "unwilling to change."

It was also a time when the medical model dominated the mental health field. Psychiatric diagnoses representing areas of pathology were given and interventions were predicated on identifying and fixing problems. An emphasis on a patient's strengths, which is a prominent feature of psychology's current landscape, was absent. When interviewing parents, I asked few, if any, questions to elicit what they perceived to be the strengths of their children or what they considered to be their own assets as parents. Relatedly, I was more apt to speak with children and adults about their problems than invite them to elaborate upon their interests and strengths.

## THE POWER OF MIND-SETS

As I worked with youngsters in a variety of settings it became apparent that to place the emphasis on pathology not only limited my appreciation of the courage and strengths of individuals, but it also impacted on and weakened my treatment approach. I became increasingly intrigued by the manner in which our perception of other people and our understanding of their behavior determined our interactions with them. I recall a meeting with several clinicians who were involved with the same family. One described the mother of the family as a "manipulator who constantly manipulates the system to obtain services" while another clinician observed this same woman as "a true advocate for her children, a mother who realizes that if you want services for your kids you have to fight for them." The first framed the mother's actions in a harshly negative way, while the second interpreted her behavior as strength. Not surprisingly, their divergent views played out in the efficacy and comfort of their meetings with her.

A concept that I began to articulate in my workshops and writings, and further refined and elaborated in collaboration with my colleague Dr. Sam Goldstein, was that of "mind-sets" (Brooks & Goldstein, 2001, 2004, 2007; Goldstein & Brooks, 2007). We defined mind-sets as assumptions and expectations we possess about ourselves and others that guide our behavior. We may not even be aware of certain assumptions, but they influence our actions.

For example, a teacher may be angry with a child without fully realizing that the anger is rooted in the teacher's assumption that the child's constant asking of questions is an intentional ploy to distract the class. In addition, the teacher may not be aware that his anger is not as disguised as he believes and is being communicated through facial expressions and tone of voice.

In contrast, another teacher with the same child may assume that the child's ongoing questions represent an attempt to understand the material being presented. This teacher is less likely to express negative verbal and nonverbal messages and more likely to win the child's trust and cooperation by offering assistance, perceiving the child as feeling vulnerable rather than being oppositional.

### A Challenging Position: A Beginning Change in Mind-Sets

A pivotal shift in my mind-set from a focus on pathology to a strengths-based perspective occurred in 1973 when I assumed perhaps the most challenging position of my career, as principal of the school in a locked door unit of the child and adolescent program at McLean Hospital, a psychiatric facility outside Boston. Within several months I began to feel disillusioned, frustrated, angry, and burned out. My response as well as that of my staff to the angry youth in our program was to become increasingly rule-bound, controlling, and punitive. These inpatient youth reacted to our misguided disciplinary techniques not by becoming more cooperative but with a greater resolve to disobey.

I frequently think about my initial experiences at McLean Hospital. At the time I did not give thought to the ways in which my assumptions about the children were contributing to an approach that actually increased their anger. To be honest, I did not view the assumptions as assumptions but rather as the "truth." What did I see as the truth? If someone would have interviewed me in 1973 and asked, "Describe the kids in your school?" I would not be joking if I answered, "I think they're out to get me and my staff. I think they plot every night on the inpatient unit about how to make our lives miserable."

If someone would have asked, "You have children in your unit between 5 to 16 years of age, what kind of future do you predict they will have?" I would have responded, "It would not surprise me if by the time they are 18 years old many of them will have hurt themselves or others, many will be heavily into drugs, and others will probably be in jail."

I am convinced that on some level the children and adolescents "read" our mind-sets, especially as our assumptions found expression in our daily negative interactions with them. Feelings and thoughts such as I had cannot be easily disguised.

I will never forget the day when one student, who continuously found his way to the "quiet room," defiantly said to me, "You don't get it, do you Dr. Brooks?"

"Get what?" I responded.

"We are going to outlast you."

Comments such as these eventually prompted the realization that if we continued to apply the same approach with these youngsters that had proven patently unsuccessful, we would continue to encourage the very behaviors we wished to stop. Consequently and wisely, we adopted a different outlook that contributed to the implementation of more effective strategies. Little did I know at the time that within this new perspective was housed the foundation for what was to become the direction and passion of my career, namely, the desire to nurture hope and resilience in children. I was beginning to shift the spotlight from examining and exposing what was wrong with the students in our inpatient unit to highlighting their strengths.

Let me share a couple of examples. I discovered that some students changed their stance from resistant to cooperative based upon the words and tone of voice I used. They were more likely to follow my request when I said, "I need your help," as opposed to my telling them what they had to do. For instance, to counter an ongoing problem with vandalism, we asked students to join staff as members of a "space committee" whose responsibility it was to notify me of any graffiti or damage and offer suggestions for a cleaner physical plant.

Initially, a few staff questioned whether the inclusion of students on the "space committee" would encourage more vandalism with one predicting, "The kids will do more damage so they can write a longer list of repairs." This dire prediction did not turn out to be the case. Vandalism was reduced significantly. One student said to me, reflecting an increased sense of ownership and responsibility, "It's our space and we have to keep it clean." This was the same child who just several weeks earlier I had viewed as destructive.

A second illustration of a shift in mind-set concerned Billy, a nine-year-old boy hospitalized for aggressive outbursts and "sadistic behaviors," including killing small animals. Billy was adopted at birth and several months prior to his hospitalization his adoptive parents gave guardianship back to the state since they could no longer handle his outbursts. In essence, Billy came to believe that two sets of parents had abandoned him, his biological parents and his adoptive parents. His mind-set was dominated by strong beliefs that others could not be trusted and that their intention was to harm him. These beliefs fueled intense anger that was not easily modulated given his learning and language delays.

Each of Billy's first two days at our school lasted only a few minutes. Upon entering the classroom, he quickly picked up a chair and threw it at one of his teachers. This resulted in his being sent back to the inpatient unit, spending much time in the quiet room as a result of his escalating angry outbursts. At a staff meeting called to discuss how best to handle Billy, the conversation initially centered on the most effective ways of punishing him. We all agreed that we could not permit a child to throw chairs or attempt to injure others. But as the discussion progressed, I had this nagging thought that six months from now we would still be considering more punitive measures to curtail Billy's violent acts.

One of our teaching staff offered an insight that when first stated met with incredulous stares from colleagues, including myself. What prompted these stares was a very simple comment, but one that was to have a far-reaching impact. In considering Billy's behavior, she observed, "I think one of his problems is that he is programmed to throw chairs."

She could see the quizzical expressions on our faces and explained, "Billy doesn't trust people. He doesn't want to be in school. Based on the records we have, school has been very difficult for him. He becomes easily frustrated and angry and the only way he knows how to deal with these intense feelings is through aggressive behaviors. It is as if he is programmed to act this way since he doesn't have any alternative behaviors available at this point."

After absorbing her comment I had an epiphany, which may sound so obvious but was not at the time. I thought, "If Billy is programmed to throw chairs, there are others who are as rigidly programmed as he is, namely, myself and the staff. As soon as he engages in his predictable behavior, we engage in ours. We restrain him and place him in the quiet room."

I shared this insight with the staff, emphasizing that I was not blaming any of us nor was I implying that Billy's behavior should not be met with consequences. However, what I was suggesting was that if we were to create any possibility of altering Billy's programmed behavior we had the responsibility of changing our programmed reaction.

Although I said I was not blaming us for Billy's behavior, several staff wondered if I was. One asked, "Are you saying that if the behavior of a kid in our school doesn't improve, it's our fault?"

I clarified, "I'm not saying it's our fault. What I am saying is that if what we are doing to manage a kid's behavior is not working then we have a responsibility for thinking about and applying different strategies. Otherwise I think the kids in our school will continue to act the way they have been acting, which hasn't made any of us very happy."

After a thoughtful discussion, the staff agreed that we should consider a different approach with Billy. We concluded that a change in our behavior would only be effective if we shifted our mind-set from seeing Billy as an angry, violent child to viewing him as a needy child who had experienced little, if any, success in his life and had difficulty trusting others. We were aware that if we were to short circuit Billy's intense programmed behaviors, we had to do something he was not anticipating, something that would surprise or startle him. We also brainstormed how to use his feelings of emotional hunger and neediness in a constructive way so that he might allow others to enter his world and demonstrate their capacity to nurture and care for him. The staff devised a creative, thinking-outside-of-the-box strategy guided by a strengths-based vision.

The next day I stood at the entrance of the school. Just as Billy was coming in, most likely prepared to throw another chair, I looked at the woods that faced the school and said in a loud voice, "We have a big problem at McLean." As we had hoped, Billy appeared startled by what I said and glanced at the woods with an expression of bewilderment.

"What's the problem?" he asked.

I responded, "You have a room to sleep in at McLean, I have a home to go to after I leave work, but all of the birds at McLean Hospital are homeless, we don't have one birdhouse on the grounds of the hospital."

My pronouncement about homeless birds had as one goal diverting Billy's attention from throwing chairs. In addition, the content of my message represented an attempt to capture through the use of metaphors what we believed were Billy's feelings of homelessness and a lack of belonging. We wanted to find a productive outlet for his sense of neediness by providing him with an opportunity to feed others, anticipating that this action would lessen his anger and his violence directed toward both humans and animals. While this was our hope, we were not certain of the outcome of our intervention.

Billy's response to my proclaiming the existence of homeless birds further reinforced my belief in a strengths-based approach. He immediately said that we had to do something about this problem and we should build a birdhouse. With the assistance of his two teachers, the ones at whom he had thrown chairs, he was engaged in planning and building a birdhouse. He became involved in reading about birds and how to construct a birdhouse, measuring dimensions, buying wood, accepting help while doing the building, waiting a day for the paint to dry, making a peanut butter ball with seeds as food for the birds, and then placing the birdhouse on a tree near the entrance of the school.

The birdhouse project accomplished several key goals. For a child accustomed to failure, it invited him to demonstrate mastery and competence and then to feel comfortable in displaying his finished product for all to see and admire. For a child hesitant to read or engage in learning, it provided the motivation to discover the benefits of taking in and then applying new information. Almost every phase of the project required Billy to learn to plan and to delay action, not an easy undertaking for such an impulsive child. Very importantly, for a child who was suspicious and always seemed in an attack mode, the task established opportunities for him to relate in a trusting and cooperative spirit with others.

I will never forget the look and smile on Billy's face as the birdhouse was nailed on the tree and staff and children praised his finished product. I will never forget my thought that prior to the birdhouse activity his provocative actions during his brief first two days at school had prompted us to see him as a violent, not very likeable child with whom it was difficult to connect. We now viewed him as a child in pain and realized that if we were to decrease his anger we first had to lessen his pain and provide him with opportunities to display his strengths and experience a sense of dignity. After the birdhouse project, Billy's outbursts diminished noticeably both in terms of frequency and intensity. His relationship with his teachers and other students showed significant improvement.

I believe that I learned more from Billy and many other children and adolescents in that inpatient unit than they learned from me—even from the boy who threatened, "We will outlast you." They prompted me to appreciate and learn about their inner world, to reevaluate my goals and interventions, and to replenish my own life with greater purpose and passion. David Crenshaw (2008) expressed similar feelings when he poignantly observed:

> I feel honored and privileged that my life work entails listening to the stories of countless children; children whose narratives call out for understanding; children whose pain requires witnessing; children who long to unburden; and whose voices need to be heard. It is the sensitive and delicate work of empathic and relationship healing of the wounded spirits of our children. I feel so fortunate; I can't imagine a calling more rewarding or meaningful. (p. 141)

## MIND-SETS THAT HEAL AND ENRICH THE LIVES OF CHILDREN

In considering the power of mind-sets, I began to grapple with a question that I have raised in many of my workshops and writings, namely, "What is the mind-set of a parent or professional who touches the mind, heart, soul, and spirit of children?" In my presentations for mental health professionals and educators I have posed the question in the following way: "Assume you were charged with the responsibility of developing a curriculum to train both future and/or seasoned professionals to be as effective as possible with children. In addition to insuring that the curriculum includes the technical skills necessary for their roles, what other material would you include in order to insure that the mind-sets they develop results in their enriching the lives of the youth they serve?"

This is more than just an academic question. If we can define the features of the mind-set of professionals who are effective in interacting with children, especially youngsters who have experienced inordinate emotional hurt and pain, we will be in a better position to train all professionals to embrace this mind-set and the interventions that flow from it.

Based on my conversations with countless children as well as the adults in their lives, I believe there are several key assumptions that comprise the mind-set of effective professionals. While I believe most professionals subscribe to these assumptions, I think it is essential not only to identify them, but to keep them in constant view so that they may serve as guideposts in our work. I also advocate that professionals engage in ongoing dialogue with colleagues about the assumptions and expectations that determine the basis of their interventions with children. Such dialogue will increase the likelihood that all members of a staff share a common treatment philosophy and approach.

The following are a selection of those assumptions that I believe are essential ingredients of the mind-set we should adopt:

## Children Have the Capacity to Overcome Adversity and Become Resilient: The Significance of a "Charismatic Adult"

As noted earlier, initially I was very discouraged as principal of the school for inpatients at McLean Hospital's child and adolescent program. I did not entertain thoughts of a promising future for the children in my care. I did not envision them as rising above their current problems.

In the years since 1973, my own experiences as well as burgeoning research in the field have taught me that no child should be written off, that youngsters possess an impressive ability to overcome significant obstacles, that resilience represents what Ann Masten (2001) refers to as "ordinary magic." During the past 15 to 20 years there has been increased interest in attempting to identify those factors that help children to cope more effectively with adversity and demonstrate resilience (Brooks, 1994; Brooks & Goldstein, 2001; Crenshaw, 2008; Goldstein & Brooks, 2005; Katz, 1997; Luthar, 2003; Werner & Smith, 1992).

I learned firsthand that children can sense when we have lost faith in them (and ourselves). Thus, it is essential for professionals to know that a consistent finding in the resilience literature is that one adult can alter a child's life forever. We must never forget that resilience is rooted in the relationship that children experience with caring adults. Julius Segal (1988) captured the immensity of this relationship when he wrote:

> From studies conducted around the world, researchers have distilled a number of factors that enable such children of misfortune to beat the heavy odds

> against them. One factor turns out to be the presence in their lives of a "charismatic adult"—a person with whom they can identify and from whom they gather strength. (p. 3)

While Segal highlighted the role of teachers as charismatic adults, the label can be affixed to any adult who nurtures hope and optimism in children. To serve as a charismatic adult, we must truly believe in the fortitude and persistence of children to become more optimistic and resilient. We must also understand that while many wounded, mistrustful youth may attempt to provoke and push us away, we must not be deterred. We must remain at their sides and help them to understand that we will not abandon our mission to enhance their lives and to have them experience us as caring adults. I learned the importance of this mission from Billy as well as from many other boys and girls with whom I interacted at McLean Hospital and in my clinical practice.

## All Children Are Motivated from Birth to Learn and to Be Successful

I have been dismayed at many clinical or educational meetings when someone questions a child's motivation to learn or to confront different tasks and challenges. I believe that when an adult uses words such as "unmotivated" and "lazy" to describe a child, it is an indication that the adult's view of the child is dominated by a negative mind-set. These are accusatory words that in essence blame the child. It is important to recall the writings of the late Harvard psychologist Robert White who expressed the belief that there is an inborn drive in children to succeed at tasks and to master their environment (White, 1959).

When I have espoused White's position at clinical meetings or in my workshops, some have countered by offering examples of children who do not seem interested in succeeding, but instead run from tasks or sabotage our efforts to assist them. As a therapist I have found it beneficial to understand these seemingly self-defeating behaviors as desperate attempts on the part of these children to avoid situations that they believe will eventuate in further failure, disappointment, and emotional distress. Why attempt a task if you judge it is beyond your capacity to succeed? Why invite a person into your life whom you believe might display behaviors similar to others in the past who have emotionally or physically abused or abandoned you?

If we subscribe to the proposition that all children wish to be successful and that their avoidance behavior is an expression of their fears and hurts, then instead of labeling them as "lazy" or "unmotivated," we can raise the question, "What can I do to lessen their fears and heal their wounds?" Time and energy directed toward answering this last question frees us from resorting to accusations and provides an opportunity for the emergence of strengths-based, creative therapeutic strategies.

## All Children Have "Islands of Competence" that We Must Identify and Nurture

If we are to avoid falling into a trap in which we resort to judgment, accusation, and a focus on pathology, we must give more than lip service to spotlighting a child's strengths. We must actively identify and reinforce these assets. Years ago, while reflecting upon the self-doubts and low self-esteem displayed by many of my patients, I had an image. I recall thinking that many of my patients appeared to be swimming, or perhaps drowning, in an ocean of self-perceived inadequacy. To counteract this image of despair and pain, I thought of another metaphor, one that reflected strength and accomplishment. It was at that point that I began to say that every child (and adult) possesses at least one small "island of competence," one area that is, or has the potential to be, a source of pride and achievement.

This metaphor represents a symbol of hope and resilience, constantly reminding me that all children have strengths. Those of us raising or working with youngsters have the responsibility of locating and building on these islands so that eventually they will become more prominent than any existing ocean of inadequacy. As I began to focus on and reinforce the strengths of children, I discovered that a "ripple effect" occurred, in which they were more willing to venture forth and confront situations that had been problematic for them.

In my meetings with parents and teachers, I immediately ask them to describe the strengths of their child or student. I also ask children what they perceive as their own strengths and if they say, "I don't know," I respond, "That's okay, it's something for us to figure out." Once islands of competence are identified, I consider the various ways they can be used as part of our treatment plan.

For instance, when I asked Larry, a 10-year-old angry boy who disliked school, what was it that he enjoyed doing and what was it that he thought he did very well, he responded that he loved to take care of his pet dog. His happiness and excitement were immediately apparent as he described how best to care for dogs. I mentioned Larry's island of competence to the principal who was very receptive to offering him the position of "pet monitor." The principal asked Larry to come to see him. At the meeting he asked Larry to become the "pet monitor" of the school and handed him a laminated "union card" with the words "pet monitor union" and Larry's name on it. The principal explained that to begin with, Larry would be expected to arrive at school 10 minutes early each day to take care of a rabbit that one of the classrooms had recently purchased.

Larry handled his duties in a very responsible manner, in marked contrast to his history with school requirements. Within a short time, the principal entrusted him to take care of other pets. Larry's teacher approached him and said she was very impressed with his knowledge of pets and encouraged him to write a manual about animal care that could be placed in the school library. Larry had always been reluctant to write given his learning problems and he informed his teacher that he didn't like to write. She responded that she knew he and some other students did not enjoy writing, but that she would assist him. Larry wrote the manual with his teacher's help and it was bound and added to the library. In addition, by the end of the year he "lectured" in every classroom in the building about taking care of pets.

Larry's aggressive outbursts and his resistance to doing school tasks decreased noticeably after he assumed the pet monitor position—a position in which he was given the opportunity to display and be acknowledged for his strengths.

A charismatic adult recognizes that a strengths-based approach requires us to identify and call upon a child's islands of competence. Such an approach also directs us to teach children to appreciate that mistakes are *expected* and *accepted,* and that mistakes and setbacks can provide information for future success.

### Empathy Is One of Our Most Significant Skills in Permitting Us to Look Beyond the Overt Behavior of Children and Understand Their Inner World of Emotions

I have frequently stated that one of the most basic skills for enriching any relationship is empathy or the ability to see the world through the eyes of the other person. Daniel Goleman (1995, 2006) has highlighted empathy as a significant feature of both emotional and social intelligence.

To be a charismatic adult, one must be empathic. Such adults constantly engage in self-reflective questions, including (Brooks, 1991; Brooks & Goldstein, 2001):

"What words do I hope children use to describe me?"
"What have I done in the past few months so that they are likely to use these words?"
"What words do I think they will actually use?"
"How certain am I of what words they would actually use? Have I built into my interactions with children ways of obtaining feedback from them?"

I have encouraged caregivers to actively seek feedback and gather information from children that will assist us in understanding how they perceive us. I have found that the very act of securing feedback from children contributes to their feeling that we care about them. The following are several examples:

There are teachers who have asked students to complete anonymous questionnaires about what they like about the teacher and the class and what they would change.

I met a teacher who developed with students a one-page "report card" that they completed on him during the four times a year when he gave them their report cards.

We developed a questionnaire at McLean Hospital that was completed by both children and their parents following a meeting in which a psychologist and educator reviewed test findings with them. The feedback we obtained focused not only on specific test scores and their implications, but in addition, how caring and thoughtful the professionals were perceived to be and whether they encouraged and spent adequate time answering questions. We discovered that a couple of well-meaning staff members were often seen as being rushed and using too much jargon that they did not explain. The feedback we provided to these staff was very helpful in their modifying the ways in which they translated test findings and related to the children and their parents.

### Stories and Metaphors Provide Access to the World of Children, Allowing Us to Be More Compassionate and Empathic

Similar to the experiences of David Crenshaw and other clinicians, I discovered that storytelling and metaphors offer a rich avenue through which to gain entry to the world of children; upon entering, we have the opportunity to learn about their strengths, coping strategies, fears, and vulnerabilities. In addition, stories and metaphors represent an invaluable format for communicating with children so that we might nurture their feelings of security, hope, and resilience (Brooks, 1981, 1985, 1987).

In the 1970s I read Gardner's (1971, 1975) accounts of his Mutual Storytelling Technique and became even more convinced of the therapeutic impact of stories and metaphors. Eventually, I developed my own storytelling technique that I called Creative Characters (Brooks, 1981). I found that within the first couple of sessions of therapy, children often provided metaphors that I could use to highlight key goals of treatment and begin the therapeutic process. In describing the therapeutic use of metaphors, I noted (Brooks, 1985):

> While the question of whether or not the patient is aware of the meaning of metaphors produced in therapy is important, it seems secondary to the challenge for the therapist of selecting those metaphors that will have special

> meaning for and positive impact on the patient. Preferentially, the metaphors should be those first used by the patient, but a therapist tuned into a patient's inner world can introduce metaphors that will immediately communicate a rich level of understanding. (p. 765)

Milton Erickson, one of the most brilliant and creative clinicians in introducing metaphors and stories in the treatment of patients of all ages, advocated that one need not feel compelled to move from the metaphor to the patient's "real-world" for the therapeutic effect to be felt. Jay Haley (1973), in describing Erickson's work, observed:

> Although Erickson communicates with patients in metaphor, what most clearly distinguishes him from other therapists is his unwillingness to interpret to people what their metaphors mean. He does not translate "unconscious" communications into conscious form. Whatever the patient says in metaphoric form Erickson responds in kind. By parables, by interpersonal action, and by directives, he works within the metaphor to bring about change. He seems to feel that the depth and swiftness of that change can be prevented if the person suffers a translation in the communication. (pp. 28–29)

The following are two illustrations of the use of metaphors within a strengths-based therapeutic approach.

### *Don't Push on a Grasshopper: Using a Child's Metaphors to Articulate Treatment Goals and Facilitate the Therapeutic Process*

Meredith, a six-year-old girl, was referred to me because of oppositional behavior and temper tantrums. She told me during our first session that she liked grasshoppers, adding, "You have to treat them nicely and not press on them too hard or they won't feel like jumping."

As might seem apparent, I viewed her warning about how to treat grasshoppers as a message to me about how I planned to relate to her. She appeared to be asking whether I would attempt to push her too vigorously and, if I did, she would refuse to cooperate with me. Accordingly, I responded in the following manner (I am offering our interaction in dialogue format so that I can more easily share with the reader the rationale and treatment goals behind my statements):

> *Dr. B*: Do grasshoppers want to learn to jump? (To assess her wish to learn and grow)
>
> *M*: Yes.
>
> *Dr. B*: Do they need help in learning to jump? (To assess whether she feels others can be helpful)
>
> *M*: Yes.

*Dr. B*: Who can help them?

*M*: The trainer. (An apparent therapist figure)

*Dr. B*: How does the trainer do that?

*M*: He pushes them.

*Dr. B*: Does he ever push them too hard? (This was based on Meredith's initial comment)

*M*: Sometimes.

*Dr. B*: Why? (To determine whether she experienced the pushing too hard as an intentional and/or angry act)

*M*: I don't know.

*Dr. B*: Do you think the trainer wants to push down too hard on the grasshopper?

*M*: Some trainers might, some trainers are mean. ("Mean" was a word that Meredith used to describe her teacher, a woman who Meredith did not like.)

*Dr. B*: How come?

*M*: I'm not sure.

*Dr. B*: Gee, you really know a lot about grasshoppers so I'm wondering how would a grasshopper let her trainer know if the trainer was pushing too hard? (I wanted to introduce the notion that Meredith should assume some responsibility and ownership for offering feedback; a sense of ownership is an important feature of resilience.)

*M*: The grasshopper just wouldn't jump. (An oppositional way of coping)

*Dr. B*: Anything else?

*M*: The grasshopper could jump in the wrong direction. (Another oppositional way of coping)

*Dr. B*: Would the trainer know why the grasshopper wasn't jumping or was jumping in the wrong direction? (Similar to a previous comment, I wanted to reinforce Meredith's responsibility for what transpired in therapy and to encourage Meredith to communicate her feelings.)

*M*: No.

*Dr. B*: Hmm. That's a problem. If a trainer really wanted to help and was pushing too hard but didn't know it, he couldn't be helpful and the grasshopper couldn't learn. (In part, I was attempting to highlight the self-defeating nature of the grasshopper's coping strategies and to communicate that the trainer could be of help.)

*M*: Yeah.

*Dr. B*: That's a problem that needs solving. (I have found that an important message to communicate is that problems can be solved, another significant component of resilience.)

*M*: Yeah.

Given Meredith's interest in this dialogue, I introduced the idea of making up a story about a grasshopper who came to a trainer to learn to jump far and straight. This strategy was predicated on the Creative Characters technique (Brooks, 1981). In the subsequent weeks Meredith, through the grasshopper figure, learned important lessons rooted in a strengths-based perspective, including ways of approaching challenging tasks, requesting help, giving feedback, and coping more effectively with frustration. Her introduction of the grasshopper metaphor served as a jumping-off point, enabling me to understand significant details of her inner world and to communicate important therapeutic messages.

### *The Elephant Who Was Afraid to Try: Storytelling as a Technique to Help a Child to Become More Resilient*

Timmy, age nine, had a history of a seizure disorder since he was four years old accompanied by many developmental and learning problems. Timmy's parents and teacher reported that his typical response to a new task was to refuse to do it and say "no." Given Timmy's many developmental issues, one could easily expend much time and energy classifying all of his difficulties and lose sight of his strengths. Initially, his parents and teacher, feeling very discouraged by Timmy's lack of progress and seeming disinterest in any activity, had difficulty identifying his islands of competence.

In therapy, Timmy was initially very quiet and reticent and when he did engage in play, there was little focus to his material. Play might take the form of darts being shot wildly or paper being scribbled upon. His attention was limited and he frequently failed to respond to any of my inquiries. I recall wondering what activity I might introduce that would not only help Timmy to become more organized but also provide insight into his inner world.

Finally, an opportunity arose. Timmy in one of his rare communications mentioned that he saw a circus on television and liked the elephant act. When I asked what part he especially liked, he mentioned when the elephants walked on their hind legs while placing their front legs on the back of the elephant ahead of them. Timmy could not elaborate what it was that he liked about this procession. I was intrigued that his favorite part of the show involved the elephants balancing on two feet, especially given his history of falling down from seizures.

I told Timmy that I also liked elephants and wanted to tell him a story about an elephant. Unlike with some other patients, I felt that given Timmy's cognitive and language lags, it would be best if I initiated the story. I informed Timmy that I was going to play an elephant who wanted to join the circus, but he had to learn to walk on two legs if he were to be in the performance. I added that the elephant's name was "Johnny Scared, the Young Elephant" and that it was given that name since he was afraid he would fall if he attempted to walk on two legs.

Timmy looked relatively amused as I made believe I was trying to walk on two legs but kept falling over (a behavior that represented Timmy's falling to the ground when he had a seizure). Each time I fell I moaned, "I can't take it anymore and I'm going to quit. I'll never learn to stand on my own two feet." Upon uttering these words, I often crawled on all "four feet" behind the chair in my office and said I would never try anything else again, that it's just too hard.

In the Creative Characters technique I typically incorporate a therapist figure within the story (in the previous case example, Meredith herself paved the way for the inclusion of such a figure when she mentioned a trainer who could teach a grasshopper to jump far). I introduced a therapist character in the story I created with Timmy in the person of an animal trainer who was knowledgeable about scared elephants. My goal was to create an individual who would embody a strengths-based approach; he would be empathic to Johnny Scared's plight, help him gain the courage to face rather than flee from his problems, and provide strategies by which he could experience a sense of accomplishment. The inclusion of the animal trainer was facilitated by Timmy's interest in the story and his desire to see Johnny Scared learn to walk on his two feet.

In my use of storytelling, I have been impressed with the eagerness with which most youngsters want to play the therapist figure. I think that for many youngsters it permits them to become active problem-solvers rather than passively accepting their condition. In addition, the demeanor they display as a therapist (e.g., shouting or encouraging, being punitive or supportive) provides a reflection of how they view me and serves as a catalyst for changes I might have to initiate to strengthen the therapeutic alliance.

I invited Timmy to assume the role of this animal trainer. Much to my delight Timmy accepted this invitation with much enthusiasm and I was impressed with the focus and attention he displayed. As the animal trainer he gave me directions about walking on two feet, but I continued to fall over and moan and groan, threatening to quit. However, Timmy persisted in encouraging me as I modeled his typical form of coping (i.e., not trying or quitting).

Another figure I often introduce in Creative Characters is that of a newscaster or narrator who, within the confines of the story, can ask questions, clarify issues, and summarize themes. I have found that children are more likely to respond to questions and observations if they come from a character within the story than if I ask them the same questions as the therapist outside the story line. In Timmy's case, I portrayed a newspaperman who was covering the circus and interviewing different acts. In one sequence I played both Johnny Scared and the reporter. As Johnny Scared I informed the reporter how I had never been able to do things very well and how I always wanted to quit. Johnny said in a despairing voice, "What's the use of trying to do something if you know you can't do it."

I then responded as the newspaperman, "I can understand wanting to quit if you feel like you can't do something, but if you always quit you'll never know whether you could have done certain things. I think you should ask for help from the animal trainer."

I felt that Timmy was ready to begin to consider more effective ways of handling his struggles. I looked at him and asked as Johnny Scared, "What should I tell the reporter, does it help me when I quit?"

Without hesitation Timmy as the animal trainer replied, "Tell him 'no, it doesn't help.'"

I responded as the reporter, "Then you and the animal trainer have to figure out how to walk on two legs even if you fall down a lot."

This story lasted for many sessions. Eventually, Timmy, assuming more and more of the role of Johnny Scared, learned to walk on his two feet and became part of the circus show. As the animal trainer I applauded his perseverance and courage. At the same time we were involved with the circus story, I noticed another change. Timmy appeared more willing to respond to questions about his experiences in school. Consequently, I decided to offer some initial comparisons between his not wanting to do certain tasks in school with the predicament that Johnny Scared had faced. As I noted earlier in describing Erickson's philosophy, I don't think it is necessary to tie a story in therapy to the "real world" since I believe on some level children do so themselves. However, Timmy seemed motivated to make the connection.

Timmy's teacher reported that he was attempting more tasks at school and had written in a notebook, "Don't Quit." This was a significant occurrence since as part of the Johnny Scared theme we had hung a sign in my office with the words, "Don't Quit."

Timmy celebrated his emerging strength and resilience by requesting in one of the final weeks of the Creative Characters story that we change Johnny Scared's name to Johnny Brave.

I have learned that if we are to serve as sources of strength in the lives of children, we must look beyond their overt behaviors and search for the feelings and thoughts that trigger these behaviors. Empathy is a powerful instrument in accomplishing this task, while stories and metaphors are rich sources of information.

## To Engage Children in Helping Others

In this chapter I have described several examples in which children were enlisted to help others, whether participating on the "Space Committee" or building a birdhouse, or becoming a "pet monitor." I frequently request my patients to write stories about challenges they have faced that I can read to other patients or at my workshops. The knowledge that their story will be shared with others heightens their motivation and self-dignity. I am continuously impressed by the therapeutic benefits of what I call "contributory activities." The experience of making a positive difference in the lives of others serves as a powerful antidote to feelings of defeat, anger, and despair (Brooks, 2002). As Emmy Werner (1993) captured in her longitudinal research about resilience:

> Self-esteem and self-efficacy also grew when youngsters took on a responsible position commensurate with their ability, whether it was part-time work, managing the household when a parent was incapacitated, or, most often, caring for younger siblings. At some point in their young lives, usually in middle childhood and adolescence, the youngsters who grew into resilient adults were required to carry out some socially desirable task to prevent others in the family, neighborhood, or community from experiencing distress or discomfort. (p. 511)

Relatedly, when I was gathering material for my book *The Self-Esteem Teacher,* I requested approximately 1,500 adults to complete an anonymous questionnaire (Brooks, 1991). The first question asked them to report on a positive memory of school when they were students, something an educator said or did that boosted their self-esteem. The most cited positive memories pertained to being asked to help out in some fashion. The following are a few examples:

> "I remember when a teacher asked me to pass out the milk and straws."
> "I felt so good when a teacher asked me to tutor a younger child."
> "I remember when a teacher told me I was a good artist and asked me to draw some signs as part of an anti-litter campaign."

The positive outcome of "contributory activities" extends throughout our adult lives as well (Brooks & Goldstein, 2004). Research clearly indicates that elderly people who are involved in assisting others lead longer, more satisfying lives, even controlling for such factors as exercise and diet.

What I find distressing is when opportunities to help others have been denied to children who would benefit immeasurably from the experience. In my consultations to schools and day and residential treatment programs I have heard the following comments in response to my suggestions that certain youth be asked to assist others:

"No, they don't deserve it. They first have to demonstrate that they can handle responsibilities for their own lives before we'll let them help others."

"Why should we allow students who aren't doing their own work to help others? Doesn't it communicate to them that you will be rewarded if you fail to meet your responsibilities?"

While on the surface these kinds of reactions may seem reasonable, I have found that they are counterproductive, especially for vulnerable students. I believe that all too often the cart is placed in front of the horse. Basically, the message is: "If you first demonstrate that you can act dignified and responsible, we will then allow you to participate in dignified activities such as helping others." Many of the suffering children I have worked with feel hopeless and they don't trust us or don't trust themselves. In response to preconditions that we establish before we will allow them to engage in "contributory activities," they basically tell us to "shove off" (that would be a mildly worded reply).

My position is that if we are to assume the role of charismatic adults and soothe the wounds of children who are in pain, we must provide opportunities for these children to help others without their having to "prove" themselves first. I have discovered that when we allow vulnerable, hopeless, often angry youth to engage in activities that involve enhancing the lives of others, and do not set preconditions in which they must first prove themselves, almost all rise to the occasion. Participation in contributory activities sends a powerful message to these youngsters, namely, "Because you are on this earth, this earth is a better place."

I have received reports from many professionals, who instead of punishing challenging youth modified their own perspective and sought ways in which these youth could have a positive influence on others. One assistant principal asked an elementary school boy who demonstrated violent outbursts to assist the two school custodians each day to help clean up the cafeteria after lunch. She emphasized that the custodians, both men, could really use his help. This provided one of the few opportunities for this child to assist others as well as to interact with men; the latter was important since he was being raised by a single mother and had few, if any, male models in his life. The boy's behavior improved markedly, the result of an assistant principal who wisely avoided focusing on punishment and, instead, created an activity that bolstered the boy's sense of self-worth.

Flynn Corson, the dean of students at the Pacific Buddhist Academy in Honolulu, heard me speak, and applied the metaphors of "islands of competence" and "contributory activities" with an adolescent girl at his school. I was very impressed with the courage he and his colleagues displayed in altering their approach to this adolescent.

The girl was in the tenth grade and Flynn noted that she barely passed her freshman year, even with "an enormous amount of help from one of her teachers." He added that at the beginning of the year she was not handing in her work "and to avoid the anxiety of having to face teachers under these circumstances, began retreating regularly to the nurse's office because she 'didn't feel well.'" Flynn surmised, "I don't think these illnesses were completely feigned. When I would check in on her she would look sick, overwhelmed, exhausted. Because her grades and attendance were so low the administration began discussing the potential for dismissal."

Flynn decided to design a program for this challenging student that was rooted in a strengths-based framework. His creativity reinforced my belief that most youngsters will become more responsible if we establish a platform on which they can display their competencies and their capacity for caring. Flynn wrote, "I asked my fellow administrators to roll the dice and allow me to set up an 'internship' for this student. She really likes little kids and is a very talented musician (ukulele) and artist. I know this because I asked her what she liked. They allowed me to make arrangements with our elementary school that she could spend approximately five hours per day in various classrooms as a TA (teaching assistant). She plans lessons and implements them for first-grade math, spelling, and social studies, and fourth-grade music; she helps with the clerical work in the room and is an aide in PE, art, and the library. She has a total of 60 students in grades pre-K through fourth.

Flynn and his colleagues added another component to this girl's program that proved very successful. Flynn explained, "An interesting component of this internship is the fact we decided to maintain her enrollment in the online math program that all of our students are part of, but appointed one of our seniors to be her 'math tutor.' This means that when she's not a 14-year-old elementary school teacher, she's the student of a high school senior with the distanced oversight of the math department head.

"She's made more progress in math in the past semester than she did in her first year and a half that she was in our school. She feels that she's done this on her own. Her math mentor loves that she feels this way, and has recently approached me about starting a peer tutoring center (a work in progress)."

I was drawn to the words "she feels that she's done this on her own." This kind of attitude is a basic ingredient of a resilient mind-set (Brooks & Goldstein, 2001). In our therapeutic and educational endeavors with children and adolescents it is imperative that we encourage them to assume ownership for both their successes and setbacks in order that they learn from both.

Flynn's closing observations capture the key messages I have attempted to convey in this chapter. "She's discovered accountability and takes this seriously. I think she is benefiting most from a support team of individuals that cares about her: her internees, her math mentor, her parents, her doctor, and I are all in close touch. She has learned a lot about different learning styles as well as different instructional approaches to reach a diverse group of learners. I think this has taught her a lot about herself. She is more socially successful, more confident, happier, more organized and responsible. Our work is not done with this girl, but we have made some great progress this semester.

"More important is the fact that this situation has helped the school better define the type of institution it is. We're now more capable of taking risks to teach our kids and it seems that our student body and parents have a new appreciation for the type of commitment we're willing to make."

It is interesting how much we learn about ourselves and the values that direct our lives by the manner in which we reach out to children in our care. If we profess that we wish to soothe the hurts of children, we must act accordingly as Flynn and his colleagues did.

## CONCLUDING THOUGHT

In echoing the sentiments of David Crenshaw, I believe that those of us who work with children are afforded a great privilege, namely, to serve as "charismatic adults" from whom these children "gather strength" (Segal, 1988). If we establish as a goal the nurturing of a "resilient mind-set" in youngsters, we will be better equipped to examine our own mind-set and assumptions and develop strengths-based interventions. Such interventions can be applied to heal the pain of suffering youth, replacing their anger and despair with realistic hope and accomplishment. If we do so, we will not only have given a lifelong gift to future generations, but we will have added meaning and purpose to our own lives.

## REFERENCES

Brooks, R. (1981). Creative Characters: A technique in child therapy. *Psychotherapy: Theory, Research and Practice, 18,* 131–139.

Brooks, R. (1985). The beginning sessions of child therapy: Of messages and metaphors. *Psychotherapy, 22,* 761–769.

Brooks, R. (1987). Storytelling and the therapeutic process for children with learning disabilities. *Journal of Learning Disabilities, 20,* 546–500.

Brooks, R. (1991). *The self-esteem teacher.* Loveland, OH: Treehaus Communications.

Brooks, R. (1994). Children at-risk: Fostering resilience and hope. *American Journal of Orthopsychiatry, 64,* 545–553.

Brooks, R. (2002). Creating nurturing classroom environments: Fostering hope and resilience as an antidote to violence. In S. Brock, P. Lazarus, & S. Jimerson (Eds.), *Best practices in school crisis prevention and intervention* (pp. 67–93). Bethesda, MD: NASP Publications.

Brooks, R., & Goldstein, S. (2001). *Raising resilient children*. New York: McGraw-Hill.

Brooks, R., & Goldstein, S. (2004). *The power of resilience: Achieving balance, confidence, and personal strength in your life*. New York: McGraw-Hill.

Brooks, R., & Goldstein, S. (2007). *Raising a self-disciplined child*. New York: McGraw-Hill.

Crenshaw, D. A. (Ed.). (2008). *Child and adolescent psychotherapy: Wounded spirits and healing paths*. New York: Jason Aronson.

Gardner, R. (1971). *Therapeutic communication with children: The Mutual Storytelling Technique*. New York: Science House.

Gardner, R. (1975). *Psychotherapeutic approaches to the resistant child*. New York: Aronson.

Goldstein, S., & Brooks, R. (Eds.). (2005). *Handbook of resilience in children*. New York: Springer.

Goldstein, S., & Brooks, R. (2007). *Understanding and managing children's classroom behavior: Creating sustainable, resilient schools*. New York: John Wiley & Sons.

Goleman, D. (1995). *Emotional intelligence*. New York: Bantam.

Goleman, D. (2006). *Social intelligence*. New York: Bantam.

Haley, J. (1973). *Uncommon therapy: The psychiatric techniques of Milton H. Erickson*. New York: Norton.

Katz, M. (1997). *On playing a poor hand well: Insights from the lives of those who have overcome childhood risks and adversities*. New York: Norton.

Luthar, S. S. (Ed.). (2003). *Resilience and vulnerability: Adaptation in the context of childhood adversities*. New York: Cambridge University Press.

Masten, A. S. (2001). Ordinary magic: Resilience processes in development. *American Psychologist, 36*, 227–238.

Segal, J. (1988). Teachers have enormous power in affecting a child's self-esteem. *Brown University Child Behavior and Development Newsletter, 10*, 1–3.

Werner, E. (1993). Risk, resilience, and recovery: Perspectives from the Kauai Longitudinal Study. *Development and Psychopathology, 3*, 503–515.

Werner, E., & Smith, R. (1992). *Overcoming the odds: High risk children from birth to adulthood*. Ithaca, NY: Cornell University Press.

White, R. (1959). Motivation reconsidered: The concept of competence. *Psychological Review, 66*, 297–333.

# 3

# Reverence for Spirituality in the Healing Process

*James Garbarino*

Reverence and spirituality are naturally linked. When stripped of theological concepts, when encountered at its core, religion is about reverence and spirituality if it is about anything. Of course, many religious traditions and institutions lose their way on this point, becoming diverted by "worldly" concerns of institutionalization, material accumulation, partisan judgment, and power assertion. Thus, there are "religiously oriented" approaches to therapy, but they often get off track when it comes to reverence for spirituality. But if we confine ourselves to the core of reverence and spirituality, whether it comes in religious garb or not, we naturally ask, how then does this translate to the healing process?

I believe it is an important aspect of what differentiates "healing" from "treatment." Few practitioners have articulated this as well as Rachel Naomi Remen (2006) in her book *Kitchen Table Wisdom: Stories that Heal*. A physician who has spent decades becoming a deeply wise and kind healer, Remen lays out the many ways in which healing is rooted in reverence and spirituality. She says, for example, "People who are physicians have been trained to believe that it is a scientific objectivity that makes them most effective in the their efforts to understand and resolve the pain others bring to them, and a mental distance that protects them from becoming wounded by this difficult work. . . . Yet objectivity makes us far more vulnerable emotionally than compassion or a simple humanity. . . . Inner peace is certainly the ultimate resource for those dealing with suffering on a daily basis. But this isn't something achieved by distancing your self from the suffering around you. Inner peace is more a question of cultivating perspective, meaning and wisdom even as life touches you with its pain. It is more a spiritual quality than a mental quality" (pp. 78–79).

I believe this conception of the relationship between reverence and spirituality in the process of healing flows directly from an expanded conception of what it means to "know." How do we know what we need to know about the human experience? I start from a belief that there are three principal paths to understanding: science and humanities, subjective human studies, and soul searching. Each is a way of trying to know, a process rather than an event. A complete understanding requires all three: healing demands it.

Let me give an example of how these three ways of knowing coexist in the real world, an example that mirrors the issues we face in life as a whole. Consider children in therapy. The outcome of the therapy hinges on the skill of the "players," as well as random, perhaps unmeasured or even unmeasurable variations in child(ren) and therapist. So where do the three ways of knowing come into it?

The science of the treatment hinges on the fact that the link between the skill of the "players" and the outcome is neither fixed nor completely random. In this, the treatment situation mirrors human life in many important aspects. For example, the odds that a child will develop conduct disorder are conditioned by gender, parental treatment, temperament, and social context. The odds are particularly large that conduct disorder will arise if a child is male, experiences child abuse, has the MAOA gene turned "off," and lives in an impoverished and socially chaotic family and neighborhood. These odds are much lower if the child is female, born into a middle-class and nurturing family living in a coherent, pro-social neighborhood. But odds only apply to large numbers of multiple events and never completely account for outcome.

From a subjective human studies perspective, the treatment process (like each of our lives) is about each participant's specific experience and what it means to that individual. The other biographical dimension of therapy lies in the fact that the significance of the experience depends upon who you are as an individual. Thus, for a child with parents who express a consistent rejection of the child, for a child of low self-esteem, or for one with intense emotional investment in holding a grudge against the world, the treatment process may be thwarted by the meaning of "behaving well" to the child. It's a matter of understanding the child's story fully.

Each of us has a personal story. These stories are particular to our "luck" from day to day and year to year, our talents and abilities and how our environment welcomes or rejects them, and how we respond to these events to create our emergent stories. For example, some poor children in abusive families who carry with them vulnerable temperaments defy the statistical odds of their situation: some well-cared-for children with access to many external and internal resources fall into chronic patterns of antisocial behavior. Whatever it is, each individual's story is a unique expression of how they encounter and experience life.

What about soul searching? From a deep perspective, the treatment process is at best an imperfect exercise in the critical business of spiritual enlightenment. While in general, life may be more comfortable with treatment success that leads to "social competence" and "social acceptance," soul searching reveals that if the process of obtaining or having any form of worldly success distracts from enlightenment and love it is a dangerous delusion. For example, a deep understanding of trauma reveals that it can teach a great deal about the meaning of life and is not just "pathology" to be corrected and cured. Treatment can harness this understanding so as to help the client develop a bigger and deeper connection to the life of the spirit. Indeed, if we define trauma as the simultaneous experience of overwhelming negative cognitions and overwhelming negative arousal we must acknowledge the fact that it has a positive twin (overwhelming *positive* cognitions and overwhelming *positive* arousal), that we might call "transformational grace."

The arousal and the cognitions are only experiences, after all, and as such "only" material, as are everything material that does not nourish the spiritual. Once again, this mirrors human life in general. From the perspective of spirit, for example, how long you live is not the issue, but always "how well." I thought of this in October 2002, when I was asked to deliver a talk at a church in Virginia at the time that the "Beltway Sniper" was at large—shooting at random people in the area of the church.

I recall the conference organizers' concerns that attendance would be down because of people's fears of going out in public and thus exposing themselves to the shooter. I remember the palpable anxiety as my host and his family exited their minivan and walked from the parking lot to the church building. As I stood at the pulpit I spoke of the irony of this situation. Certainly one of the core beliefs of Christianity is that you must always be ready for death by living a life of faith. Jesus spoke of this, saying, "I am the resurrection and the life. Those who believe in me, even though they die, will live" (John 11:25).

It is a testament to the difficulty of living completely in congruence with our spiritual beliefs that the many Christians attending the conference found it impossible to live as their faith instructed them to do. Living the life guided by the spirit is easy in the abstract, but difficult in the reality of day-to-day life.

The issue is always how you live the time you have, not defined by conventional, material "outcome measures," but rather by progress toward spiritual enlightenment. In the fall of 2005, two deaths occurred in my social world within the space of one week's time. The first was my 88-year-old mentor, Urie Bronfenbrenner, who died after a life of enormous worldly accomplishment and family proliferation (5 children, 16 grandchildren, and 2 great-grandchildren). The second was a 10-year-old boy in my church who died after living most of his life with cancer. To all who knew him, the little boy's life was completely fulfilled spiritually, even while it was grievously abbreviated as a biography and was a physical catastrophe in scientific, objective terms.

Ironically, a long life of public accomplishment, even a life of public service as an academic, does not necessarily equate to a life of spiritual growth. Rachel Remen offers a compelling example that many a distinguished professional might identify with. In *Kitchen Table Wisdom* there is a short vignette about an eminent academic physician she heard lecture 45 years ago when she was a medical student. At his retirement dinner he gave a talk. She writes, "People had come from all over the world to honor him. It was a memorable evening. The talk he gave was memorable too . . . an intellectual tour de force and he received a standing ovation. Later in the evening a group of medical students went to speak to him and . . . One of our numbers asked him if he had any words for us at the beginning of our careers, anything he thought we should know. He hesitated. But then he told us that despite his professional success and recognition he felt he knew nothing more about life now than he had at the beginning. That he was no wiser. His face became withdrawn, even sad. 'It has slipped through my fingers,' he said" (pp. 205–206).

In the eternal world of the spirit, our time on Earth is a very minor matter, made significant only by virtue of the fact that it affects our opportunities to engage the universe and progress toward enlightenment. By all accounts, the little boy with cancer lived a very "spiritually efficient" life in the sense that he achieved a rare level of consciousness and closeness to God in the few years of life on Earth available to him. No one would invite cancer into the life of child just to create the opportunity for spiritual growth and consciousness, of course, but there is no denying that ultimately it is the spiritual "accomplishments" of living that matter most. In this same way, the experience of dealing with challenge and threat can lead to spiritual growth *if* the process of treatment becomes one of healing, *if* the agenda is driven by the goal of spiritual growth and enlightenment. Reverence for spirituality is at the core of all this. Again, Rachel Remen expresses this well: "People who have sought healing everywhere else are often afraid to look within, afraid to find, at depth someone insignificant or even unworthy. Yet this is rarely the case. The soul is our birthright. At depth, everyone is beautiful. Often it is the discovery of the 'spot of grace' that heralds the beginning of out deepest healing" (p. 262).

Science and humanities is the domain of academics. Here we find the efforts of scientists and humanists. The former (both physical and social scientists) seek to demonstrate the objective empirical realities of human behavior, growth, the latter look for patterns in culture and history by analyzing literature and other human documents.

The goal of the scientists is to document empirical patterns, statistical relationships, and predictive and verifiable hypotheses concerning the objective features of human development. The science of treatment is a matter of documenting correlations between therapist behavior and child client outcomes. The humanists seek to tease out of documents such as therapy transcripts larger patterns and themes of meaning.

Whether they are scientists or humanists, this is the predominant discourse in academic pursuit and policymaking. It is the world of "on average" and "in general" and "on the whole" and "most" and "few" and "many." Both science and humanities have at their core a set of rules and principles to govern the pursuit of knowledge and its communication to others. In this sense both are "objective." This is not to say that biases don't creep into the process. They do. But the intellectual beauty of science and humanities is that there are well-established tactics and strategies for exposing and disposing of these infringements upon the fundamental commitment to objectivity when they are detected.

But while science and the humanities map the large-scale psychological, sociological, biological, cultural, and demographic terrain of human development and child therapy, this alone does not lead us to the end of the journey. Set within this conception of life is the individual experience of being human—and adult therapist or a child client—which inescapably leads us to a second methodology, the study of subjectivity in what some scholars have called human studies.

Human studies is the study of the unique meaning that individuals recognize in themselves, and the processes and strategies for communicating that meaning to others, albeit inadequately. There are an enormous number of specific influences on any single individual human being, influences which interact and accumulate to produce very different end results. Therefore, no two human beings share exactly the same life pathway, no two of us have exactly the same autobiography. And no two people have the exact same experience of therapy.

There are general commonalities, to be sure, and these are the object of study by science and humanities—for example, in the psychological study of "treatment efficacy." And there are points of perfect intersection between separate lives, the points at which two individuals recognize that despite the myriad of differences that differentiate them as people there is a point of complete correspondence. Some of these moments are illustrated in Bruno Bettelheim and Alvin Rosenberg's excellent book on child therapy, *The Art of the Obvious.*

But subjective human studies recognize that each individual life is unique in the experiencing of it. It asks us to try to walk miles in the shoes of another human being. But even as it asks us to adopt this strategy for feeling what the other feels—empathy—it recognizes that whatever we learn will be intrinsically and inevitably incomplete and approximate. This differentiates human studies from science and humanities, where precision rules.

Subjective human studies demands that we allow room for a process that moves beyond the constraints of a purely academic focus on objectivity and verification. It demands that we allow for subjective information to become a valid vehicle for understanding developmental issues. Human studies focuses on the narrative accounts of subjective experience, on therapy as the illumination of life stories, as the improvement of autobiography in ways that lead to changes in behavior.

It's about discovering and assessing the meaning of human experience as it is lived and understood by a specific individual in a specific situation—the child in therapy. It's about human beings in their singularity as represented through the stories these human beings employ to make sense of themselves as individuals (and as members of groups). Human studies are the documentation of identity: It is each of us telling the story of my life. It's the study of biography.

Human studies seeks to illuminate subjectivity while acknowledging that any such effort can only be partial, no matter how long we work at it and how smart we are. It recognizes that no matter how good the story, how poignant and evocative the language of that story, and how diligent the listener's efforts, there is always loss of validity from the teller of the story to the listener. What we learn from the creating and telling of our life stories advances our understanding of the human experience. But it too is incomplete.

In other words, empathy is never complete. In human studies you can never know exactly what I experience unlike in science where, when I say the temperature of this liquid is 45 degrees Fahrenheit you can know exactly what that means and exactly replicate my data. Philosophers of science have called this phenomenon of you knowing what I know (and I knowing what you know) "intersubjective transmissibility."

All human communication is ultimately imperfect, thus intersubjective transmissibility is always and inevitably partial and incomplete. But even were it to be complete, it would not be the whole human story because human beings are more than the story of moving their bodies around on the planet Earth. Human beings are spiritual beings, and this requires yet another kind of knowing.

This third form of human study is soul searching. Here the goal is to make and sustain contact with human spiritual realities beyond the facts of physical experience, and even the individual's subjective account. And, like science and humanities, there is a defining methodology to soul searching.

What is this method? It is contemplation, meditation, and prayer. It is what Zen Buddhists like Thich Nhat Hanh call "mindfulness," the practice of paying attention to reality "in the present moment." It is to sit quietly for a long time and focus your attention—perhaps through observing your breathing or through meditative prayer. The evidence is clear that if you follow this methodology you will reach approximately the same conclusions. In this sense, then, science and humanities share with soul searching the goal of documenting and illuminating common realities, while human studies seeks to document and illuminate particular realities.

In the case of soul searching, these common and "objective" conclusions find expression in statements such as these three: "there is more to life than the material experience of it" and "love is the fundamental imperative of the universe" and "peace comes from caring without attachment and desire." When child therapy becomes healing, helping a child understand, embody, and live by these principles becomes the goal and the rationale for the process, treating it with reverence the principal criterion for evaluation.

Apply the method and you reach the three basic data of soul searching, just as if you embrace the methodology of science and direct your attention to human biology you almost inevitably come to the conclusion that the current form of human bodies is the product of evolution—despite the claims of "creationism" or "intelligent design." Similarly, whether you are the Christians St. Ignatius of Loyola or Mother Theresa, or the Buddhists Thich Nhat Hanh or the Dalai Lama, the common method leads to the same essential results, although how you express these truths and what implications you draw for day-to-day living in the specific cultural and historical context of your life may vary.

Some Native American cultures speak of "soul traveling" as a way to integrate the experience of body/mind/brain/soul. Christian, Jewish, and Muslim mystics see the path in prayer. Buddhists and Hindus speak of insight meditation. This approach starts from the reality of human beings as spiritual beings having a physical experience, and proceeds from there. Does anything in human experience really mean anything beyond what individuals, groups, and cultures say it means? Is there anything more than psychology, biology, sociology, and anthropology on the one hand, and history and literature on the other? Without soul searching, the answer is "no." With soul searching the answer is "yes."

If we do not recognize the spiritual realities underlying the literary realities of narrative accounts and the statistical descriptions of empirical realities of the social and physical sciences there is only one empirical reality—"You are born. You live. You die."—and only two basic narrative accounts: "I am born. I have a nice day. Then I die." or "I am born. My life sucks. Then I die." If this is all there is, the therapist is limited to damage control (when life really does suck, as it does for so many children) or persuasion (when the material conditions of a child's life really are pretty good and it is just a matter of replacing "negative attribution bias" and "negative social cognition" with improved reality testing). But to go beyond this in the face of profound loss, trauma, deprivation, injustice, harm, and horror requires a move beyond therapy to spiritually grounded healing.

Only soul searching can expand an afflicted child's life stories by integrating them into the eternal realities of spirituality. Buddhism and Christianity offer elaborate worldviews that transcend the experience of conventional life and place the individual in the realm of the timeless, where oneness with the universe becomes "obvious." You can't go there without this spiritual practice (but limiting yourself to the theology and practice of conventional religion may not take you there either).

Human beings are spiritual beings and thus have spiritual needs. No simply material conception of human identity will suffice. This is a vitally important recognition for understanding the quality of the world inside and outside the child treatment setting. To recognize a child's spiritual needs is to recognize that he or she has a fundamental need to know that he or she lives in a meaningful universe, that there is something more to his or her life than the material experience of those lives. And it means that the healer recognizes that he or she is fundamentally the same as the child client!

All civilizations have many texts to guide us in this effort. I think some of the best of them come from the Sermon on the Mount. In Matthew, chapter 5, the words of Jesus are recorded thus, "Blessed are the meek for they shall inherit the earth." On the face of it, this may be the most ludicrous truth in the Bible. It is ludicrous because even a superficial look around at the world seems to make the idea that the meek shall inherit the earth improbable in the extreme. Any abused and traumatized child can attest to this. This is true, except for the protected spiritual spaces in our lives, such as in church on Sunday mornings, in the synagogue on Saturdays, in the mosque on Fridays, and in the Buddhist meditation room any day of the week, when it seems easy to believe. Ludicrous yes in the everyday material world, but true none the less, because a deeper analysis reveals this to be a profound insight.

A pastor friend much more knowledgeable than I tells me that "meek" here means "those who have the strength to be gentle." Those who have the strength to be gentle in the face of the material and warring world as it is—often cold, hard, and violent—reach a state of spiritual enlightenment, and nothing is more precious than the bliss and peace this brings. And no one needs it more than the traumatized, abused, deprived child in therapy.

Enlightenment does not come automatically to children. Children are not always automatically exempt from the temptations of hatred. When I visited Croatia during the tail end of their war with Serbia, an 11-year-old boy said of his Serbian enemies: "They are monsters and I hope our army kills them all as they deserve." It doesn't take much imagination to understand how he learned this lesson from the adults in his world, parents, teachers, neighbors, relatives, and politicians.

The Dalai Lama teaches that compassion is more than a feeling dependent upon the sympathetic nature of the other. It is the ability to remain fixed on caring for the other person regardless of what that person does, not just out of sympathy for the other person but from the recognition that it is best for ourselves to live in a state of compassion rather than hatred. It flows from a kind of spiritual intelligence, which "knows" that reverence of life is the prime directive of the spiritual life, and the mark of the healer.

## REFERENCES

Remen, R. N. (2006). *Kitchen table wisdom: Stories that heal.* New York: Penguin Group.

# 4

# Reverencing the Many Faces of Each

*E. Mark Stern*

The head is like the sky. Always turning around and around inside.

—Paul Bowles, *The Sheltering Sky*

## CARNAVALE

There we were my wife and I, lost in any known direction on the edge of Saint Mark's Square in the City of Venice. The vaporetto (water bus) had taken us to what, in time of Carnavale, may possibly be the most crowded hub of the Western universe. Boarding the canal vehicle steps away from the hurry-shaped exit of the train station, there was the sensation of a massive stampede—people of all ages, speckled and strewn with the vulgarity/seductiveness of zealous travelers in conflagrations of costumes and masks. These days abutting on Lent were atmospheric ecstasy!

As we wedged our way through the walkways and corridors, crossing over footbridges and fluttering mounds of confetti, Virginia and I savored a bubbling eternity of the adrift. Carrying our suitcases through the directionlessness of amassments of revelers, we were curiously lost both for want of our hotel and a creeping exaltation at being jostled into ultimate anonymity. Tall and short, coupled, tripled and singles, tots and elders—each and all costumed as gracious Marcheses and Marchesas, plundering pirates, clockwork buffoons, valiant knights and cherry-cheeked maidens, and, in a foreground of their own, there were squabbling children, most adorned with multicolored three-pointed jingling headgear (*liliripes*), their slightly older siblings toting scepters (*marottes*), such as those etched on medallions of the later Roman Empire. Rococo assortments of twosomes, many whose couturier skills were breathtaking, were willingly coaxed into posing for cacophonies of snap shooters. The universal traffic of humanity stampeding Saint Mark's Square was fraught with trickery and notorious abandonment, and as Shakespeare described: "a villain with a smiling cheek."

Masquerading has long been a venerable Venetian tradition. Since the 13th century, citizens of Venice would, with the sleight of a facial mask, awaken the mystery of transformation. Citizens of past centuries celebrated their clandestine conspicuousness between St. Stephen's Day (the day following Christmas), until the stroke of midnight on Shrove Tuesday which signaled the beginning of Lent. There were even those who began to don their masks earlier, from Ascension, early in October, to Christmas. Being masked for Venetians, past and present, has afforded them a jumbling range of chosen, but no less necessary, personal identities.

Carnavale, while hardly the travelogue of this chapter, testifies to the astonishing transformative potential of each person who seeks to be appreciated within the focus of psychotherapy. Over the decades, I have come to see the psychotherapeutic arena, especially the one that fits into the rubric of "humanistic," as a marching parade of transforming and transformative facial bearings and carriages. These presentations, rather than mocking stability, in fact, remain faithful to the scope and variety that each person is both destined and free to be.

As the sights of Carnavale loom in and out of vision, the desire to venerate, to revere and to sanctify the sweeping array of what it is to be person, create the foundations for the mission of being and doing psychotherapy.

## AN EVOLUTION OF MASKS

The art of doing psychotherapy is taught on many levels. My own good fortune is to sense that "little red thread" of imparted information. Much has come about through an extensive range of mythology, fiction, painting and sculpture, mixed media, and a readiness to see within the lingering echoes that occur when least expected. Here the lessons come about as they portray perfusions of transformative capacities and prospects.

And so, when my two older children were in grade school, but close to the time my son was to be born, it was my unexpected good fortune to attend a one-man performance by a traditional Indonesian Pemia mask maker. As introduction to his presentation, he explained that, in his culture, ancestral ceremonial masks were the necessary ingredients of "second funerals." These ceremonials traditionally occur after some time period has elapsed since the death of a tribal member. On a selected day, the corpse is dug up and masks fitted to adorn the remains. Such facial funeral masks are of a flat and oval design, composed of light wood carved and painted with extended noses and overridden by horizontally shaped eyes and double-arched brows. Multicolored jewels are imbedded, signifying the caste the individual belonged to.

Over much time, the tradition of the Indonesian mask maker has evolved from dressing the dead into a new into a living performance art. My having had the privilege of watching the presentation of the man, whose name has longed skipped my memory, continues to unfold the transformative possibilities of the assent of relational psychotherapy. He brought a myriad assortment of facial masks, all conforming in shape to the traditional pattern. Yet each depicted differing faces rooted in the Indonesian—a giant Komodo dragon lizard, a brilliantly plumaged bird of paradise, a human dwarf, a fierce Sumatran tiger, and an elderly priestess. This range of representative beings, each one with a mask depicted by the traditional shaping of features served as launchings into much more. As the mask maker adorned a particular face cover with one hand, his entire being magically conformed to the distinctive characteristic set into mask. Literally, the mask maker, evolved for the one designated to adorn the death remains of the ancestor and endow it with new life, at this moment delineated with his trunk, limbs, and torso the animating ebb and flow of each of the creatures. The transformative fermentation of the mask maker's body leapt into a dramatic empowerment well beyond the boundaries of the ceremonial mask. Yet the alternating masks served as sparks bestowing each with spontaneous life, enticing with crowned counterstrokes—all became extensions of the particular mask he was adorned with.

As I gazed at the spectacle in a small lecture hall, I experienced something of what the young Sigmund Freud might have gone through in 1885 as he observed the Jean-Martin Charcot demonstration of the hypnosis of a hysteric woman at the Salpetriere Hospital in Paris. For me, the transformative link between mask and life force made an impression that has continued to inspire my own work with psychotherapy clients. Each person is invariably endowed with a capacity to adorn his or her being with variable mantles of being. This capacity for variation, when realized, enlarges the means of emotional sustenance. Likewise, being more than one appears to be, reaffirms the magnitude of potentialities.

## PERMUTATIONS

In my 60 years of psychological practice, I have witnessed and revered profound alternations in the repository of people's resources. Rather than use actual masks, I have made abundant use of mirrors and self-imagery (Stern, 1964). Witnessing the ensuing emotional permutations has awakened much that was dormant in me. This inauguration of intersubjective transformation remains lifelong. I recall well the 30-something married women who hesitated to quite know how to identify herself whether by her maiden/professional name or the hard-to-spell many-lettered married name. As she eventually explained it: "I am, for the proximate time the name I use. Those who I first meet are surprised when I tell them about the person behind the name I may not have initially introduced myself as." Then, there was the man who could only allow his temper and anguished face to reign when exchanging words with another male. I asked him to be aware of the force behind his near rage. As he transitioned into this exercise and his facial muscles notably relaxed, I was reminded of a Cyclops's singular eye mutating into the elegance of a Monarch butterfly.

Melusina, who, as Carl Jung (1969/1980) etches her, is, in European folklore, the elemental spirit of fresh water, seen at first with a granular tail and a flowing indeterminate shell, then, all at once, translated into a double-headed crowned person. Moving from formlessness into form (much as an optical illusion—now this and now that) offers the perspective of what I consider to be multidimensional pirouetting between appearances and potentialities. Certainly any such radical shift suggests the phenomenon of gazing on the outside as the inside likewise appears.

Transformative imagery is, in Jean Genet's telling of his thievery, moving first into his self as "master of tools" and finally as a "myself." Genet the playwright creates his many possible-identity characters propelling into "the mysterious cipher of the pure imagination, (culminating in) Genet himself" (Sartre, 1963, p. 405).

In Genet's play *The Maids*, Jean-Paul Sartre, his biographer, speculates that "the two maids (have) no other function than to be the other, to be, for the other—herself as other" (p. 617). The maids, as written into Genet's script, were boys playing the roles of the two maids, masquerading themselves in their mistress's wardrobe. Genet, a master of masks and their inevitable metamorphoses, conjures up "the child who is transformed into an alligator" in circulating ritual (pp. 4–5).

## TRANSSHAPING, EMPATHY, AND THE SOMETIME FAILURE OF MASKS

Literature is, of course, filled with surprise leading to what I see as fictional characters transshaping into new identities. Similarly, ordinary life overflows with an enormity of radical shifts from one identity sequence to another. As this chapter will demonstrate, what is termed empathy is that time when masks, that is, facial expressions, are purposely or unwittingly shared. Here a mutual bounty evolves as each slips into the other's being. Here mutating selves gather together.

Yet the mask a person wears may not truly cohere as authentic. Looking back on his childhood in London during the Second World War, a man I knew recalled that he and his schoolmates were assigned gas masks as precautions against the inevitable German air raids. The masks were made up to resemble Mickey Mouse in order to win the hearts of the children. Yet these gasmasks failed to alter the personal terrors that the youngsters bore. A dejected person advised "to put on a happy" face will inevitably sink into confusion. However convincing, there are bound to be masks, which despite their outward glimmer, can be assaulting and haunting. In Leoncavallo's opera *Paggliacci*, the clown, despite his ability to draw laughter from others, is incapable of penetrating the deep sadness occasioned by his wife's affair with a rival.

## "DEFENSES" AND COPING

Anna Freud (1985) systematically outlines character "defenses" that are, in her eyes, manifested by young people. These, she contends, are primarily bound together by psychopathologies labeled as obsessions, phobias, and hysterias. Anna Freud's psychoanalytic underpinnings are viewed by her as labor-intensive modes which aid adolescents' somewhat greater competencies in dealing with the world. From her vantage point, there are those youngsters who tend to learn to keep safe from would-be adversaries by donning an analogous behavioral uniform. She uses the example of the young child who was accidentally hit on the head by a distracted teacher. During this same child's analytic session a few days later, he appeared in a costume of armor holding a play gun and sword. The analyst concluded that the boy had decided to transform himself into a macho giant, now capable of inflicting similar punishments on others.

Certainly there was reason to conclude that this makeover from the superficially injured child to armed "thug" could lead to being a bully. Some masks may well become fixed while others linger in less obvious ways. I well recall a garrulous woman who vividly recalled being a meek 11-year-old, suddenly discovering sources of strength as she escaped from the clutches of an insidious attacker about to sexually abuse her. Weeks later when a loitering group of tyrannizing tormentors surrounded her as she was riding her bicycle, she found herself once again that strong shrewd being as she broke loose from their harassment. Then in her teen years, the essential fragility with which she tended to identify would give way to a surprising resilience when faced with formidable challenges. This mask of courage would essentially follow her into her adulthood where it served her well in her career and social relationships. When once I asked her about the "mask," she shook her head, tears flowing, "There's this source of protection that I feel that I can always count on."

I long ago had the opportunity of counseling a 12-year-old boy whose parents had been referred by a family physician. Mitchell complained of recurring "sore bellies." As we spoke, he felt undone by his mom insisting that he eat more food than he had the appetite for. His dad, in order to avoid further conflict, would bribe him to finish what was on his plate. One day Mitchell "doubled over" in great, what he called, "pretend pain," but one that freed him from further irksome obligations.

As we spoke, I took note of Mitchell's contorted lower lip. I asked him if he had ever been aware of the twisted lip. He responded by grinning, as if saying "no way." After awhile I invited him to join me in a fun experiment. Handing him a face mirror I encouraged him to make as many faces as his fancy took him. When I said the word "freeze," he was to hold his pose, whatever that be, and after studying it, give it a name. "Hum," he paused, "How 'bout Tunner the tiger?"

"Get into that face ever more," I coached.

Looking deeper, he blushed, wondering if what had been an overwhelming tiger had suddenly become a lonely "scary cat."

"With what name?"

"Zina."

"And where and how do Tunner and Zina meet?" An impish grin suddenly passed along his lips. "Freeze!" I called out. "Look as closely in the mirror as you possibly can."

There, with no small amount of amazement as he recognized his lower lip to be that point of contact between ferocious tiger and prudent kitty. It was agreed that I could help him "mask making," a transformation of his face into a blend of the fierce tiger and lap kitty. I suggested that he play into the facial mirror, moving it enough distance so that he could better see his shoulders. He hunched and released them just so. "What are you seeing?"

"I like what I see." Later: "They really look strong."

"Let's get a look at how strong they have been." He brazened his shoulders slightly upward. Then he smiled. "More like the tiger than the cat."

"You know Mitchell; I've just been realizing that tigers are great big cats. What's more, tabby cats need to see themselves as daring hunters."

A minute later he smiled, "I can imagine myself being a really shrewd, but not a spitting cat."

Our rapport had steadily ripened. Mitchell's stomach pains became more of a language. "With your decision not to spit," I surmised, "your stomach is set to rumble." With that, he set out his fingers like feline claws and opened his mouth full force. "Just testing out my spitting," he replied.

"Looks pretty much intact to me, powerful, yet strategic," I observed.

He proceeded to tell me about how his dad was always being critical of him. In order to end his day, he'd just agree with his father's displeasure, even if he was feeling that what his father complained about was "something else again." Mitchell's mom often came to his defense, hardly a way of enriching the father/son relationship. With Mom's moving in to shield Mitchell, his dad would usually take his newspaper and silently leave the room. Sometimes he'd go out for a prolonged walk. He felt sorry for his father.

"Do you feel pain for your dad whenever he cuts loose?" I asked.

"Most of the time I do, but I'm also pissed off at his starting the rampage." Nonetheless, Mitchell felt a deep closeness to his father, and I suspected that the stomach pains would often start when the going got hot and heavy. I chimed in again: "It's got to disappoint you that you can't rescue either you or him."

"Thanks," he said, "But I just wish my dad didn't always have to bust me."

"I can see what you mean on your face. Your lower lip tells much more of your discomfort than any words ever could."

During our sessions, we would sometimes play a game of chess, often as a prelude to what was currently on his mind. Not surprisingly, it was during some of these matches that I would find myself wondering why he overlooked the strategy of taking, say, a knight or in one instance my queen. Mitchell was a really bright kid, so it was becoming obvious that he was passing up on possible moves that might otherwise be obvious to him. I noticed a major facial blank as he would allow himself to cede the match to me.

I minimized commenting on attempted strategies. I did, however, remark on the passive expression that would accompany his approach to those matches which he too often lost. It was during one of my commentaries when he casually informed me that it was his dad who taught him to play when he was about five years old, but that in their matches, he had not once been able to defeat his father.

I just listened with much interest, and as I did, I felt something brewing that could hardly be ignored. "Hey Mitchell," I recall saying, "How about just trying and see yourself in the mirror, first as losing a match; then in contest as an undefeated champion." Mitchell, now quite used to my requests that he see his reflection in the mirror, was delighted to comply. Moving about, pretending to cogitate moves on an imaginary board, he first grinned nervously, and then we both noticed how all his small facial muscles gave way. His shoulders noticeably slumped and the game was "ceded."

Now it was his turn to replay the match with all the skills of a Bobby Fischer. The "game" began with a noticeable certitude. There were cheers coming from an "alter ego" as he mouthed pleasure at his "fancy footwork." Most conspicuous was the way he raised his shoulders. Then as he came in for a victory, he prompted the feline "spit" that had now become part of his emotional resources. "And now ladies and gentlemen," he announced, as if a radio commentator, "we have a new world champ—meet Mitchell." Truly a well-enacted victory coming from the depths of this youngster's soul, I applauded and yelled out "Bravo! Bravo!"

The next time we met, he eagerly looked forward to setting up the chess men. From his opening first two moves, I was in check. Soon after he had me checkmate. He said that his dad had taught him several killer opening moves. I could feel a wave of confidence that was to be solemnly revered. I rose from my chair and offered a standing ovation. We tried a return match, and he easily won again. I handed him the mirror, and decidedly there was a triumphant air of conquest. "You are relishing what you see in the mirror."

What followed was heartening. Although his dad rarely won another chess match against his son, camaraderie developed. His father researched junior memberships in a neighborhood chess club where, with the help of his dad's tutelage, he climbed in his ratings. Mitchell found a new zest. With the encouragement of his history teacher, Mitchell helped bring interested kids together in the first-ever chess club in his middle school. Mitchell's mother had some getting used to as being needed less and less as a defender of her son. I had several opportunities to hear her out, and was pleased to see her new sense of Mitchell's maturation and the resolution of his stomach aches.

Stemming from wide-ranging encouragement and reverence, Mitchell's repertoire of being was extended. Reverence and awe become manifest within the scope of ever-enriching contextual transformations. This shift of perspectives enhances who a person is, bringing to light a broader range of meaningful emotions.

## QUEST FOR IDENTITY

In all of my interactions with clients, I emphasize what it is about them that attracts my spoken and unspoken esteem for who they are, even as they themselves may yet to have located these components in their sense of themselves. Often, when contradicting feelings take hold, each one seemingly in control only to lose place to the other, I see something of what Ronald Laing (1960) refers to as the divided self. But, with contradictions seemingly prevailing, I am simply unwilling to dismiss what I consider to be feelings at variance as "mood swings." Rather, with Martin Buber, (1955, p. 96) I prefer to view such sequences as ways of "experience(ing) the other side." In line with such valuation, I see humanistic psychotherapy as an exercise in reverencing all of the client's experience (Stern, 1966).

Elsewhere I have described (Stern, 1965, pp. 294–295) a female client whose manner in therapy was to attempt to echo characteristics of mine as her way of realizing needed changes in her own life. Her phrasing and physical attitudes were somewhat carbon copies of mine. In consequence of her attempting to be like me, she, in fact, missed my real presence. Furthermore, her efforts at simulating her sense of me initially resulted in holding us in a deadlock. Given a stalemate she seized on, I followed her suggestion that we link our fingers and palms in touch as a way of fist joining, and soon gently parting as a way of appreciating our differences and that we were indeed separate selves, but very much able to be in contact with one another.

Wearing what seems to be an exact mask of the other can miss the essence of a relationship. Yet even two or more people wearing identical masks at a masked ball soon discover that distinct portraits emerge. As my client found the courage to see herself as unique, she granted herself that uniqueness which allows for distinctiveness in a crowd. As her own voice began to exfoliate, it was as if she heard and could own distinct new sounds. Carl Jung (1954, p. 285) beautifully qualifies the need to make sure that "projections" of the other do not overtake one party. If such happens, then there is no authentic relation, and so "without a relationship (that other) falls into a void." There is need to search for and to establish the identity that can be reverenced.

## ENHANCING THE COMPASS

Larry, an erstwhile client, had braved a major cloudburst in order to keep an appointment with me. The early part of his entry was spent in making it possible for him dry off, a task that required the assistance of my housekeeper. Procuring towels and robe, upping the thermostat, and placing his socks and outerwear in the dryer were prefaces to an eventual readiness to embark on his therapy session. Yet, what uncharacteristically followed was a clearing of throats accompanying some awkward pauses. When, at last, he floundered into the heartland of the session, his words bungled. It took several subsequent sessions before he was able to reflect of how his familiar "therapy mask" had been breached by the effects of the thunderstorm. According to Larry, being drenched seemed to have blocked both of us from recognizing "the strange territory" to which we each had been taken. As he saw it, a confusion of identities had taken over, only later to become grist for his mill.

Going over his sentiments, he was no longer the very self-contained client he thought he had been. Unable to take his usual cushioned seat across from me, he lost whatever perspective he had developed. He shivered and felt like a child walking round in a dream. Our conversation, which according to him, had a certain note of profundity, had suddenly shifted to a fear of being "in trouble" for which he felt an urgency to apologize. Larry was a business executive more used to hearing others apologize. Yet it was this same apologetic sense of having been troublesome which allowed for an entirely new picture of seeing a long hidden sense of personal unworthiness.

Looking at me, several sessions later, he observed "shadowy corners in your face staring at me like the grandma who beneath it all was the relentless wolf in Little Red Riding Hood."

"Perhaps the better to see you?" I deliberately proposed. The concealed predator had, after all, his marked advantages. What we were dealing with was me as grandparent, but basically inseparable from a cunning wolf.

"I guess I need to know that the wolf cares. A once fond girlfriend of mine used to oversee a restored pack of endangered wolves put in the wilderness of the West. . . . Most people see me as a not so gentle wolf. Now suddenly, I see you, my therapist, as a wolf in sheep's clothing. I feel vulnerable and at risk."

"Larry," I said, "you had spoken of your quick temper and how you thought that you'd 'inherited' it from your mom's mother who lived with you until you were about nine when she was placed in a nursing home. You loved her, and felt so safe being with her. But she had that temper that might leap out unexpectedly at you, your mom, your brother, and rarely, and with great consequence, at your father. She was a tough 'old broad,' to quote you, but a source of deep love all at the same time." Later I then recounted the fable of the banished royal twins Romulus and Remus, who were rescued from extinction as they were plucked from the river by Lupa, the archetypal she-wolf. She became their nursing mother. A cross-species that blended the unlikely. "When we initially met, you said that you were used to being in charge, and indeed, it was you who 'conducted' our sessions. I've long learned the value of needing to be with you on your terms. Somehow you were flowing fast and furiously and something needed to interfere with the tides. And suddenly you fear not being in absolute control. Beyond that, you've pinned a mask of the loving side of your grandma on my presence. You know you've done that. And then, you sense that angry wolf that can sometime be seen beneath that mask. I am exposed as the wild wolf."

Identities emerge from the groundswell of personal constructions—those we choose to adorn us and those endowed by our genetics and further convoked by family, friends, and the culture. It is up to each individual to choose or not choose to increase the range of emotional, spiritual, and social responses. Under the rubric of renewal, restoration and expansiveness, there well may be what some others see as the dysfunctional. It is often the eye of the beholder that establishes identity. It is also the beholder who has the option of reverencing the wonder of the beheld. For the humanistic psychotherapist, there remains the task of perceiving the compass and depth by which each client contracts to live. For the therapist who seeks to discern the emotional nucleus of the client, there will always be the adventure of witnessing the augmentation of contiguous essences, not as mere poses and assumptions, but as new and sometime stormy awakenings. The therapist who *beholds* in contrast to the one who tends to cast diagnostic verdicts, finds that novelty and rebirth (in whatever way) goes beyond the sometimes formulaic resources of "role playing," "modeling," or "cognitive rehearsals." The zest needed to accompany the client; to confirm benedictions on the client's new finds; to be the willing travel companion—transforms the journey from clinical task to what the French philosopher Gabriel Marcel (1964, p. 12) speaks of as "creative fidelity" in which there is the manifestation of "co-presence . . . (under the aegis of) the career of the soul." Here the therapist can appreciate what is most varietal, authentic, and special to each soul.

## REVERENCE FOR ALL MASKS

To reverence all masks is to dismiss none as counterfeits. There needs to be an affirmation of that repertoire of being, always attempting to be born and reborn; each mask must be revered as an unbroken expression of the whole.

Gaston Bachelard (1964, p. 108) writes of the birth of the being; rousing to awareness like Aphrodite stirs from her shell. Bachelard appreciates the birth of any identity as creating a necessary dialectic between ascending being and its durable foundations. In this case, no mask is ever concealment, but rather an animated representation of what is being born along with the evolution of its distinctive properties and unique delineations. Any newly revealing identity can be thought to be illusory or evasive. Its underpinnings from which it arises serve to stabilize its genesis and its potentialities.

Although the foundational shell or source is tribal or archetypal, humanistic and transpersonal psychotherapy endeavors to promote dialogue between source and expression. Yet this dialogue is bound to have paradoxical consequences. As James Hillman (1989, p. 198) cleverly puts it, "no one knows you better than your family" and "my family can't see me at all." All the same, being recognized for who one is and being less than appreciated all fit the same dilemma. Jesus, according to Biblical accounts, was hardly recognized in his own hometown. Confusion and even nonrecognition mobilize as the result of an individual pondering his or her identity: "Am I really who I presume to be or am I fighting for what my mother wanted to be herself? Am I really creative or am I merely trying to placate my father's constant criticisms of me?" It would be unusual not to be haunted by these seeming contradictions. A pioneer psychoanalyst Marion Milner, writing under the pseudonym Joanna Field (1934/1952, p. 34), looks back on her personal adventures of self-knowing: "I have often wondered whether what I have called my discoveries may be only true for me. My path may have wandered through deserted and waste places which may be quite off the main highway. . . . Certainly, however, in the later stages of what I had thought was a lonely trail I came upon the outskirts of a country which seemed to be well known to the few, though little spoken of and I think unguessed by the many."

The task of the humanistic psychotherapist is to remain companionable with each and every expression of being since all sides grace the coin, and all are to be revered as essential. To my mind, the humanistic therapist continues to remain best available in what amounts to "a relationship dedicated to heightening sensitivity to experience" (Stern, 1966, p. 286).

## SEPARATION AND REUNION

The woman who walked into my office appeared nonchalant. Vera mentioned, quite obliquely, that she had been referred by her neurologist in order to sort through ways of coping with the unpredictability of multiple sclerosis. Her eyes floundered as she spoke. From this floundering, I sensed, and as matters would have it, my instinct proved to be quite correct, that she was out to prove that nothing I might say would have any impact.

The objects around my office, though less than beguiling, would henceforth be her distractible frame of reference. Though continuing to look directly at me, she spoke mainly admirably about her father's "John Wayne looks" in comparison to my humdrum appearance. I asked if it was important that I match up to her dad's image. "Probably," she said, somewhat off-key as she next took pains to slough off the physician who referred her to me as "a wispy man" who, she proposed, probably knew less about her disease than he claimed. No matter, thought I, that this man was considered as a lead research scientist in multiple sclerosis at a top-notch medical school in New York City.

Her mother, though while living under the same roof, was reported to be virtually separated from her father. Vera said about her mother that she "sported her own hunky boyfriend," someone close to Vera's own age. Her father, too, she said offhandedly had his own assortment of "boyfriends," most of whom were young aspiring actors and fashion models. She mentioned at first that she had three siblings—a sister a year older and two brothers who were in their various stages of college. Later she denied having told me about "brothers."

On a late evening about three or four weeks into our twice-weekly sessions, I received a phone call from someone who had a shy, but quite concerned voice. She identified herself as Vera's sister, and before I could spell out the ethics of confidentiality, she quickly let me know that she didn't expect me to do any more than listen to what she had to say—which, she emphasized, would be brief and to Vera's possible advantage. The gist of her remarks was that Vera had told her that she had been lying to me. In fact, she was in a great deal of physical, but, especially, emotional pain. I thanked her for the information and ended the conversation, but not before informing her that I would need to tell Vera that, out of concern, she had phoned me with information I would then have to share.

When I next saw Vera, I opened with telling her about the phone call. She appeared less than interested. "Oh, she, Lily has an exaggerated sense of me. She can be so dramatic." She said that she had not told Lily that she had lied to me. Momentarily, I paused. I had not yet had the opportunity to tell her what her sister had said. It is not my usual practice to probe for inconsistency, but I did move the tone of the conversation to asking her to tell me more about how she and Lily, both reported to be living at home, had been bearing up with their parents. Vera had previously mentioned that she had long given up speaking to either unless spoken to first. Lily, she noted, is one of those who hardly ever leaves of her room. "What do you call it?" she quizzed me. Then, after I simply waited for her to continue, "Oh yes, she's agoraphobic. And she lives in a fantasy world, certainly not to be ever relied on to tell the truth about anyone or anything." At this point, I did fill her in on Lily's concern about her being in both emotional and physical pain.

"Hah," she said, "OK, let me tell you what's really happening. Yes, I have fleeting, but miserable pains—mostly in my calf muscles these days. Sometimes, I have a fear of not being able to swallow. Lily may be right about that. But that's hardly *my* story. I'm wondering why I no longer feel any desire. Not any desire whatever for anyone or anything." Suddenly she turned on her neurologist. "I keep seeing him, but honestly he's an absolute dud." I asked her why she continued seeing him for so serious an illness when she might get some other opinions. "How could I leave him? Epstein (she would never refer to him as doctor) is extraordinarily dependent on my seeing him. He says I'm some sort of 'test case' for him. Whatever," she sighed. "He apparently needs me in his life."

"So Vera, what I am hearing is that Dr. Epstein needs you as a patient more than you need him. Have I gotten it right?"

"Whoever said 'as a patient'?" she demanded. And, "Don't get me started on him."

"I think, Vera, it was you who have started on him, and since it was he who referred you to me, it 'started' even before we ever met. . . . You did tell me that you are without any desire. Has it always been that way?"

"Not before this damn disease. Before I was struck, I was 'campy,' fun to be around. I feel now like my guts are gone."

I decided to inquire, "Have there been stomach pains as an issue with the disease?"

Vera glared at me, "Every sort of pain."

"Then again, doctor," she said as if reminding me that she had no feelings such as satisfaction or dissatisfaction, "sounds as if you've not done your homework. Didn't Epstein tell you about my 'belly aching' to him?"

With her consent, I called Dr. Epstein. He said that he knew very little about Vera since she'd never followed through after an initial evaluation. "Vera has not been in my care. The reason I referred her to you was because I suspected a strong emotional basis."

That night, Lily called again. I could hardly make out her voice. But I did recognize the distinctive cough that Vera sounded in my office. "I'm really worried about Vera. She's stopped speaking to me. This is not good news. And she won't say anything to my parents. You know that they're infirm themselves. Besides, Vera is in love with Dr. Epstein, and fears that he'll finally let her know that there's nothing further he can offer her. You know my parents have multiple sclerosis as well." Then suddenly, our phone call abruptly ended.

Vera appeared a day later. "So I gather Lily called again. Well, it's been some week. My father had a blow-up with his latest suitor and asked my mom if they could get back together. Oh yes, her guy split for greener pastures a few weeks ago."

As far as I was concerned Vera's reality was at stake for her. I had no intention of destroying our line of communication. But honestly, I felt in a whirlwind of unrealities. To me an unreality is, though improbable, perhaps totally real. In fact, as time went along, I invited Lily's 'spirit' to attend our session. Vera was only too happy to comply. She was living in both realities—hers and what was seamlessly admitted to be her other self. Alas, I was the Epstein who she did feel needed her. I could do nothing, since I was the one holding onto the feelings she herself wished she had.

We continued to work together. We looked at her parents at once, very needy of her strength and concern. She did see them as once having been exotic, but had constructed an even more exotic life than ever they had had.

I recognized that Vera wanted me to facilitate her having feelings. I had no difficulty letting her know how unity was becoming apparent in her life. She did return to Dr. Epstein and was followed up with several trial medications. But in the end she knew it was time for her to seek worlds beyond her therapy sessions. I left the door open for her to revisit me at any time. These reunions were often filled with pain. But, important to her life, she sought friendship and romance. As it happened, there were grave disappointments. Vera was not an easy friend. Yet, through the years, she did seek out support groups and became a significant part of each group she ventured to join. I know that she ultimately considered her life having aggregate value. And the roles she was to play—those I knew about and those that passed me by, were Vera's passage to the capacity to look to the now in her life.

Vera has since passed away.

## REVERENCING THE MANY FACES OF EACH

Psychotherapy, though some would not agree, is never a warfare of wills nor a stripping away at self-presentations as if they were defenses (Reich, 1949; Horney, 1942). In assaults on self-presentations, there are battles to be won. Most often, in the grip of a psychotherapy war, for the therapist to win is for the client to lose. Personality may be strong or fragile, but always in need of honor and reverence for that fragility is essential. Masks, which may serve as a me or perhaps as another or others me's. They may be identified as part and parcel of a family history, or begin from a nowhere. Some masks may be, as novas, momentarily resilient. Others may long be cultivated from seed in new lands. There are the masks of Carnvale which, in the midst of daring celebration, are shed as Lent appears. Then consider the facades that restructure the entire body image, much like those ceremonial masks of Indonesia. Gas masks, no matter how textured with expression, can be signs of destruction. Other masks have the potential of redemption.

The variation of personal identities—of those born and created from fantasy or necessity—adhere to Erik Erikson's (1969/1993, pp. 265–266) notion of identity as being both the expression of individuality and the demands of communal culture. In whatever their manner, each mask is a becomingness, creating new personages from having the potential of influencing the establishment of other new identities.

Within my practice, each day; each client creates a reconstitution of who I am. Over the many years of my clinical practice, I have become increasingly aware that the first individual I meet with in the day is radically related to the client that closes the day. In fact, I go further. It's the first person that I ever saw in my psychotherapy practice who continues to affect my relationship with my newest client. All identities and appearances share an uncommon endowment. Egos and alter egos regularly emerge with expanding repertoires, allowing for renewed modes of contacts.

The client base that I continue to meet brims with sprouting potentialities. Reverencing the client's narration provides the therapist with an opportunity to know and be known all the more. Sharing in the dialogue walks the walk even as forks in the road are bound to make their appearances. As client and therapist amble together, each one points to novel assessments and nestling transformations.

Yet make no mistake, the road can frequently be dark. Jolts of malevolency appear to convolute the relationship. I've known moments of feeling imprisoned by the client's mayhem. Even then, new foci are inevitable callings for a deepening of the reverential attitude. Healing occurs as the many faces/masks/moods become recognized and revered as true resources for one another and for the whole. It is then that self and selves, mixing identities, incorporating dichotomies are given the breadth to exist "simultaneously as both self and world . . . all that we are related to" (Craig 2008, p. 247).

In conclusion: humanistic psychotherapy invites the masks that its clients wear and may exchange with other masks. Masks, long confused as defenses or defense mechanisms are often authentic modes of presenting oneself to the world. Some that just emerge may have long been concealed. Others may still be on the drawing board. No matter; each deserves a reverential attitude since each and all expressions of self are tangible as, knowingly or not, they daily interact as ensembles of a person's existence.

## REFERENCES

Bachelard, G. (1964). *The poetics of space* (M. Jolas, Trans.). Boston: Beacon Press.

Buber, M. (1955). *Between man and man* (R. Gregor-Smith, Trans.). Boston: Beacon Paperbacks.

Craig, E. (2008). The human and the hidden. *Humanistic Psychologist, 36*, 211–226.

Erikson, E. (1969/1993). *Gandhi's truth: On the origins of militant non-violence*. New York: W. W. Norton & Company.

Field, J. (1934/1952). *A life of one's own*. London: Virago Press.

Freud, A. (1985). *The ego and the mechanisms of defense*. New York: International Universities Press.

Hillman, J. (1989). *A blue fire*. New York: Harper & Row.

Horney, K. (1942). *Self-analysis*. New York: W. W. Norton.

Jung, C. G. (1966). *The practice of psychotherapy*. Vol. 16, *The collected works of C. G. Jung* (H. Read, M. Fordham, & G. Adler, Eds.) (2nd ed.). Princeton, NJ: Princeton University Press.

Jung, C. G. (1969/1980). *Psychology and alchemy*. London: Routledge and Kegan Paul.

Laing, R. D. (1960). *The divided self: An existential study in sanity and madness*. New York: Penguin Books.

Marcel, G. (1964). *Creative fidelity*. New York: Noonday Press.

Reich, W. (1949). *Character analysis*. New York: Farrar, Strauss, & Giroux.

Ricoeur, P. (1992). *Oneself as another* (K. Blamey, Trans.). Chicago: University of Chicago Press.

Sartre, J.-P. (1956). *Being and nothingness* (H. E. Barnes, Trans.). New York: The Philosophical Library.

Sartre, J.-P. (1963). *Saint Genet: Actor and martyr*. New York: George Braziller.

Stern, E. M. (1964). Mirror-dialogue approach to the treatment of a borderline psychosis. *The Journal of Existential Psychiatry, 4*, 207–218.

Stern, E. M. (1965). Direction for psychotherapy. *The Journal of Existentialism, 5*, 287–295.

Stern, E. M. (1966). Psychotherapy: Reverence for experience. *The Journal of Existentialism, 6*(23), 279–287.

# II

# REVERENCE FOR HEALING IN PSYCHOTHERAPY

# 5

# Resiliency-Based Approaches and the Healing Process in Play Therapy

*John W. Seymour*

Children are referred to play therapists for a wide range of concerns. Michael, age 10, was referred to the play therapist by his school counselor. While his educational testing placed him in the gifted program, he was failing every class and becoming increasingly socially withdrawn from teachers and peers. Maria, age three, was referred from a preschool program for pushing and hitting other children. Her foster parents, who were considering formal adoption, were dismayed at home by episodes in which Maria would ransack the house for several hours at a time, emptying drawers, closets, and containers and leaving the contents strewn in all directions. Brothers Jake and Al, age 11 and 9 respectively, were referred by their pediatrician for ADHD screening. In the initial assessment session, their mother reported that not only were the boys not paying attention at school, but also they were not getting along well with their classmates and there was conflict between them at home. Their parents had separated six months earlier, and their father had moved to another state and had not returned to see them. While each of these children had very different circumstances and concerns, they all had a play therapist as a partner in addressing these concerns.

Play therapists represent a number of helping professions, including counseling, family therapy, psychology, social work, and others, and all have shared, through a similar healing tradition with medical roots, the tendency to be more deficit-based, driven by the question, "What's the problem?" Earlier chapters in this book have reviewed the history and current issues of applying deficit-based treatment models. In play therapy, as in other psychotherapies, these deficit-based models have their limits. At the same time, these models also have been important resources for understanding the challenges faced in the human condition. In the cases of the children mentioned earlier, a play therapist would likely begin thinking about understanding these children from any number of perspectives or lenses: attachment theory, learned helplessness, grief work, developmental models, family structures, parenting models, educational models, trauma physiology models, and many more. Each of these lenses could provide a useful perspective, but these lenses can provide greater clarity if a strengths-based lens is added.

Consider the initial play therapy session with Michael and his mother. As the play therapist reflects on Michael's failure at school and social withdrawal, the therapist may wonder whether these referral behaviors suggest symptoms of depression. If so, the therapist might build on that possibility with a series of symptom-based questions, screening instruments, and observations in the playroom of how Michael may be exhibiting the symptoms of depression in his play. This process can lead toward therapeutic responses within the play, in working with parents, or in consulting with school personnel. This collection of data about the problem becomes the foundation of a diagnosis and treatment plan that informs further care and (to note a very practical concern) provides information needed for reports and billing third parties. For all of its efficiency, this approach can distract play therapists from alternative explanations of Michael's experiences and contribute to a narrow focus that may miss his strengths as well as resources within his family and social network that can reinforce long-term improvement. As Sam Goldstein and Robert Brooks (2006) have pointed out, "Symptom relief has simply not been synonymous with changing long-term outcome" (p. xiv). Resilience research, focusing on the intrapersonal and interpersonal dimensions of children adapting to challenges, can provide a new lens of understanding for play therapists from many approaches to incorporate a strengths-based approach to their play therapy (Seymour & Erdman, 1996).

## RECENT DEVELOPMENTS IN RESILIENCE RESEARCH AND PLAY THERAPY

In the past 30 years, there has been a rapid expansion of research on factors impacting the mental health of children. Resilience research has been one of the key areas of research, focusing on the identification of risk and protective factors that contribute to the emotional adjustment and well-being of children (Rutter, 1987, 1993, 1999, 2007; Waller, 2001; Wright & Masten, 2006). Resilience refers to "the relative resistance to psychosocial risk experiences" (Rutter, 1999, p. 119). Put another way, resilience describes "a relatively good outcome for someone despite their experience of situations that have been shown to carry a major risk for the development of psychopathology" (p. 120). Froma Walsh (2003) defines resiliency as "the ability to withstand and rebound from disruptive life challenges" (p. 399). Details on the mechanisms of these risk and protective factors have provided the basis for innovation in approaches to prevention, treatment, and policy issues in child mental health. Brooks (1994a, 1994b) has emphasized the need for a strong link between the research on children at risk and the provision of effective interventions.

Margaret O'Dougherty Wright and Ann Masten (2006) describe three "waves" of resilience research, representing development of the construct of resilience and its application to treatment and policy. The first wave was more exploratory, seeking to describe and catalog the qualities of children who by history had responded to major life challenges that can be crushing to children. This first wave of research tended to focus on resilience as a quality attributable to the individual child. While illuminating in many ways, it led some in professional circles and popular media to develop a myth of the "invulnerable child," who with near superhuman qualities could overcome any adversity. Particularly in the United States, where individualism and autonomy have been strong cultural values for many people, the "invulnerable child" myth may persist in clinical, community, and policy applications (Shapiro & Friedman, 1996). However, as Margaret Waller (2001) pointed out, "resilience is not the absence of vulnerability" (p. 292). Continued research on resilience led to a second wave that identified more complex, interactional relationships between resilient children and their social context of family and support systems. More recent third-wave resilience research has broadened the focus to include more preventative measures and more cultural factors in understanding how resilience is fostered (Johnson, 1995).

It is important to keep in mind this historical overview of resilience research when applying the findings to play therapy, avoiding the "invulnerable child" myth and understanding the complexity of individual and social factors that contribute to a child's ability to adapt when facing daunting challenges in life. When applied well to play therapy, resilience research can help identify the child's strengths, family and community resources available, and the processes of joining them in reinforcing the child's immediate ability to cope and longer-term ability to be prepared for the next life challenge. When applied in a more haphazard manner, focusing mainly on the individual child's qualities and simply wishing them well can be disrespectful of a child's pain and naïve of the child's ability to somehow overcome all obstacles on their own. Children, with their dependence on their caretakers, sensitivity to other's moods, and magical thinking, can feel shamed and blamed with a careless application of a "You can do it!" approach. David Crenshaw (2006, 2008) has described the importance of applying strengths-based approaches in ways that will not deny, minimize, or trivialize a child's suffering. As with any theoretical model, play therapy informed by resilience research will only be as effective as the quality of the therapeutic relationship and the nurturing environment of the play therapy setting.

Play therapy over the past 30 years has seen a surge of interest and growth, as mental health professionals from a number of disciplines have developed play therapy models within or alongside the historical psychotherapeutic models (Knell, 1993; Kottman, 2002; Landreth, 2002; Oaklander, 1992), developed new therapeutic models (Jernberg & Booth, 1999; O'Connor, 2000), and placed a new emphasis on describing the dynamics (Schaefer, 1993; Schaefer & Kaduson, 2006) and outcomes (Bratton & Ray, 2000; LeBlanc & Ritchie, 2001; Ray, Bratton, Rhine, & Jones, 2001) of play therapy. Other than Adlerian-based play therapy, earlier play therapy models have been more individually focused, but play therapy has expanded over the years to include several family-focused approaches, such as filial therapy (Guerney, 1991, 1997; VanFleet, 1994a, 1994b, 2000), Child Parent Relationship Therapy (Landreth & Bratton, 2006a, 2006b), ecosystemic play therapy (O'Connor, 2000), and family play therapy (Gil, 1994; Gil & Sobol, 2000; Schaefer & Carey, 1994).

In studying the therapeutic processes involved in play therapy across models, Charles Schaefer (1993) proposed fourteen "therapeutic powers of play" in a book by that name. These powers of play describe the mechanisms at work that make play beneficial for the child; these powers include overcoming resistance, communication, developing mastery, creative thinking, role-play, fantasy, metaphoric teaching, attachment formation, relationship enhancement, enjoyment, mastering developmental fears, and game play. These mechanisms provide a way for the play therapist to understand the dynamics in the play therapy session. The powers of play can provide an inside look at the dynamics of the play session, and an understanding of resilience processes can widen the play therapist's understanding by providing a look beyond the session to family and social supports for the child coping with adversity.

Play therapy models incorporating resiliency will need to develop ways within the model to address family dynamics and consultation with support systems. Family play therapy (Gil, 1994; Gil & Sobol, 2000; Schaefer & Carey, 1994; Seymour & Erdman, 1996) provides play therapy directly within the context of family therapy, where the therapist can tie the themes of play directly into work with the family. Family members may be involved directly in the play as an extension of the play with the child. Filial therapy (Guerney, 1991, 1997; VanFleet, 1994a, 1994b, 2000) and Child Parent Relationship Therapy, or CPRT (Landreth & Bratton, 2006a, 2006b), outline methods of addressing the parent-child relationship through planned interactions with the therapist and between the parent and child at home. While each approach varies from the other, they incorporate opportunities for therapists to model and encourage new skills for parents interacting with their children, extending the therapeutic powers beyond the play therapy room. Whatever the model of play therapy, resilience research can provide an added lens of understanding in determining the needs of children and their families and choosing the most appropriate course of action in play therapy.

## APPLYING RESILIENCE RESEARCH IN PLAY THERAPY

Michael Rutter (1971, 1987, 1993, 1999, and 2007) has been an important resilience researcher over the past 30 years, making major contributions to defining the key concepts, developing research models, and applying the results of research into clinical, program, and policy recommendations. In a review of recent resilience research, Rutter (1999) saw the strengths-based lens of resilience research being used in the clinical setting in two broad applications: reducing the risk factors and increasing the protective factors. Rutter drew from findings on both risk and protective factors to summarize eight resilience processes that could inform therapeutic approaches with children and their families.

### Reducing the Accumulation of Risk Factors

Rutter (1999) observed that risk factors impacting a child can be numerous at any given time, so one way resiliency could be enhanced would be by reducing the overall number of risk factors. An awareness of the complexity of factors involved is a good reminder of the limitations involved in focusing on any one factor (poverty, single-parent home, having a mental disorder diagnosis) in understanding the problem and generating solutions. Ben, age six, was referred for fighting with peers at school and being disruptive in class. In his initial play session, he worked feverishly building walls of wooden building blocks and lining the walls with small soldier figures. He was absorbed in his play, communicating a sense of urgency with the speed of his play and occasional dialogue among the soldiers: "Hurry! We have to hurry! The bad guys are coming! We have to be ready!" From interviewing Ben's mother, a picture of multiple challenges emerged for his life: the whereabouts of his father were unknown, the mother worked long hours and still they often did without the basics, their small apartment was overrun with mice and insects, and they were living in a dangerous neighborhood. While Ben's play did not provide a statistical listing of his multiple risk factors, the tone of his play clearly communicated his experience of being surrounded by challenge. Within the playroom, the therapist gave simple supportive statements, reflecting on the themes of his stories of danger and preparation. Over time, characters and themes were introduced into Ben's play that gently offered potential resources: "Can anyone help the soldiers? Can they trap the bad guys before they get to the walls?" Outside of the play therapy session, the therapist worked with Ben's mother and teacher to cultivate their understanding of Ben's experience and offer suggestions that might help reduce the overall risks that he faced, such as utilizing the resources of a neighborhood youth organization.

## Reducing the Individual Sensitivity to Environmental Risk

Rutter has documented (1987, 1999) how children, through prior experiences of adversity, can develop ineffective methods of emotional expression, communication, and problem solving. Chronic stress and trauma trigger changes in a child's neurophysiology that contribute to significant changes in a child's ability to continue to creatively adapt to adversity (Perry, 2006; Perry & Hanbrick, 2008). Combine the stress-based changes in coping with a child's cognitive developmental level, and the result can be significant distortion of views of causality (O'Connor, 2000), leading to an adult-sized sense of responsibility for what was likely a minimal or nonexistent role in creating the adversity that is so difficult for them. Beyond the layer of anxiety from the risk and trauma, this self-blame and overreaching sense of responsibility can lead to a second layer of anxiety, experienced as inadequacy.

At age three, Maria's brief life had already included exposure to drugs in utero, violence, neglect, and a series of caregivers of varying consistency before her placement with the foster parents seeking to adopt her. All of these contributed to her very distressed nervous system, demonstrated by her hyperactivity, hypersensitivity to external stimuli, sleep difficulties, and mood swings. In her first play session, she duplicated her behavior at home, going through every part of the play therapy room, emptying everything. Looking for possible purposefulness in her behavior, the therapist commented, "It looks like you are looking for something," to which Maria replied, "The baby! The baby! Where is the baby?" This led to a shared search by Maria, the therapist, and the foster mother, looking through the playroom for possible play materials that could be a baby. When several were located (including a baby doll, a doll house figure of a baby, and several small stuffed animal babies), she picked the baby doll and was elated, hugging and rocking the doll. Her tornado of behavior entering the playroom had become a centering, relaxing moment as she soothed herself through soothing the baby doll. The play therapy room would become for her a place where many searches for self-soothing were to continue during the course of her treatment. The therapist also worked with the foster family to better understand a number of ways, actively and quietly, that they could help Maria to develop self-soothing techniques to better regulate her nervous system. As Maria became more predictable in her ability to interact positively at home and with others, her family and support system responded in kind, giving Maria the assurance that she was loved, further easing her sensitivity.

## Reducing the Negative Impact of Adversity on the Individual Child

The shame and self-blame from a child's sensitivity to risk can be interpersonally reinforced by members of the child's family or social support system who in their own stress and frustration from the same risks begin to place blame on their child for causing the problems. Rutter (1999) noted that while children in the same family might face similar risks and experience similar family discord around those risks, the child with the higher risk was the one singled out as the scapegoat.

Anxiety can also enhance a child's sensitivity to environmental risk. Recent research in the neurophysiology of children has shown what a profound effect chronic stress and trauma can have on a child's nervous system in increasing anxiety (Perry, 2006; Perry & Hanbrick, 2008). The anxiety in the child can be reinforced interactionally, as the child's family and support system amplify the response by initiating anxiety-provoked behaviors that can trigger more anxiety within the child and anxiety-provoked behaviors from the child (Gil, 1994). Play therapists can often help the child's parents to shift from being more problem-focused to more solution-focused by use of reframing, showing how the child's challenging responses to adversity may also be signs of strength.

Gina, age nine, came into the play therapy room and the therapist offered a simple invitation to browse the play materials and see if she wanted to play with something. She gravitated to the doll house and proceeded to set up the people figures in different rooms and began to play out a family interaction. As she continued to play, the intensity of the play increased, and one of the child figures was told by an adult figure, "You've been bad! You have to leave!" When Gina was asked where the child figure went when she left the house, Gina responded that "She had to go to a counselor because she had been bad." The therapist then had the opportunity to explore with Gina other possibilities of the story as the doll house play continued, with Gina making the point later that some of the other family figures were really the bad ones. Later, the play therapist in working with one of Gina's parents could expand the definition of "the problem" to a less blaming, more contextual understanding, helping to take Gina out of her scapegoat role.

## Reducing Negative Chain Reactions

The reduction of negative chain reactions enhances protective processes and serves "a crucial role in the long term adverse sequelae that may stem from risk experiences" (Rutter, 1987, p. 327). These negative chain reactions, or risk chains as described by Paul Smokowski (1998), can have a ripple effect, leading to children who feel futureless (Terr, 1990), a condition described by James Garbarino (1994) as terminal thinking. More traditional, problem-focused intake interview processes can tend to reinforce this chain reaction by focusing on the "problems" of a child, leading to the child feeling judged by adults and a need to distance themselves further in an attempt to deal with the discomfort. Parents can also have this sense of being blamed for their child's problems, which can hamper their ability to emotionally connect with their child or engage in a problem-solving process to improve their circumstances. Whatever the model of play therapy, initiating the therapeutic relationship is the first major intervention in reducing the negative chains of risk. The therapist will need to have strategies for addressing these challenges in initiating a therapeutic relationship, by providing a nonblaming, safe setting for the children and parents. As a trusting and safe therapeutic relationship is developed, the therapist can offer gentle guidance in identifying and choosing coping strategies that reduce, rather than increase, the risks.

These negative chains have both intrapersonal and interpersonal components (Rutter, 1999) that may be addressed in play therapy. On the more individual level, stress creates increased anxiety, which can become overwhelming to the child, affecting concentration, mood, and rest. This has the potential to decrease the child's affective and problem-solving responses to the next adversity, leading to an even higher level of distress. In addressing the family component of these negative chains, interventions from strategic and structural family therapy approaches can introduce change to the parent-child interactions, disrupting the negative chain (Seymour & Erdman, 1996). A highly stressed parent who sees his or her child as irritating, demanding, or controlling can benefit from reframing by the play therapist that would help the parent see the child's behaviors as signaling anxiousness and a need for reassurance.

In the earlier example of Jake and Al, who were referred for ADHD screening because they weren't paying attention at school, additional details at the intake focused on the challenges that the boys and mom had faced in response to the father and mother separating six months earlier, with the father moving to another state and not returning to see the boys. The boys' grief was palpable, and the mother alternated between being numb at one moment and irritable with the boys the next. What emerged was a pattern of the boys' grief triggering anxious behaviors that in turn would trigger responses from an overwhelmed, grieving mother that to the boys sounded irritable. This triggered more anxiousness in the boys, who would further act out, which to the mother served as confirmation that she was doing poorly in her parenting. Formerly close parent-child bonds had become stressed, with all of them becoming distracted in their grief and attempting to adjust to the loss. The play therapist initiated simple interactive games with the boys and then included the mother, helping to remind them of previous positive connections damaged by the grief and laying the groundwork for a colleague to begin a series of filial play therapy sessions (VanFleet, 1994a, 1994b), providing the mother with support and encouragement in reconnecting with the boys. As their relationships improved, the boys' inattentiveness and impulsivity were reduced and the original ADHD screening referral rationale was dismissed in favor of a grief adjustment rationale for their behavior.

## Increasing Positive Chain Reactions

Positive chain reactions that enhance resilience aim at reinforcing self-esteem and self-efficacy (Rutter, 1987, 1999; Quinton & Rutter, 1988). The referral problems that bring children to the play therapist almost always involve a combination of some disruption of relationships and a fading sense of accomplishment regarding some life task. For the individuals in the family, this often means discovering or rediscovering strengths and talents in each person and assisting them in investing in activities that build confidence and mastery, as well as connecting with members of their family and support system that encourage them in these tasks. The play therapist working with the family has the opportunity to model simple methods of communication, cooperation, and problem solving and then practice them in session.

With Jake, Al, and their mother, puppet play was one method useful in reinforcing these positive chains. In a variation of puppet play described by Eliana Gil (1994), when the family would come in with new conflict around family rules or routines, family members were asked to choose a puppet and show the therapist how the disagreement occurred. This allowed each of them to effectively communicate the details of the experience with less conflict in session, since after all it was the puppets, not the family, in conflict. The puppet play gave them the opportunity to express their feelings about the conflict, get some perspective of the other's experience, and rehearse alternatives with the puppets on how to resolve the conflict. Game playing was also helpful for this family in practicing positive relational and problem-solving tasks. With their work in filial therapy, many of these changes were successfully implemented into their home routine.

## Opening up Opportunities and Maximizing Turning Points

As children and family members develop more success in developing strengths in session, the focus turns outward to help them apply these strengths in their home and community. While adversity can bring people into greater connection with their support systems, ongoing adversity can become isolating. It is important for children and parents to be able to identify trusting and positive resources in their environment that can increase their range of positive experiences and broaden their social contacts (Rutter, 1987; Webb, 1999). Helping children develop skills in choosing positive peer relationships, cultivating better family relationships, and developing mentoring relationships are important steps to help them connect to supportive relationships around them.

Play therapy sessions, with the development of a therapeutic relationship, and with the new perspectives gained through creative play, provide the child and family with building blocks of experience that become the foundation for developing more positive and supportive interactions in their community. Taking a more systemic view of the problem and solution helps to neutralize the risk for the child and family and can give them more flexibility in adapting to future risk (Walsh, 2002, 2003).

With Jake and Al, their family had become more isolated after their father left the home. With limited time, energy, and money, they had not played their usual team sports during the last season and as a family they had not been as active in school, community, or extended family events. Over time, they set goals with the therapist for reconnecting with some of these activities and identifying others of interest that could be done on a limited budget. This allowed them to identify some new activities that they were interested in that were not shared by their father. New talents and new opportunities to relate to positive adults and peers were identified.

## Fostering Neutralizing/Compensating Experiences

As Rutter (1999) points out, while positive experiences alone are of limited benefit, neutralizing experiences can be more beneficial. Children who have positive supportive relationships with parents, extended family, school personnel, or youth mentors in the community all have a greater ability to respond favorably to adversity, particularly if those relationships provide a needed contrast to relationships that have been less trustful and more damaging.

For Jake and Al, it was not enough to simply get them signed up for more activities to fill their week. They needed activities that would give them consistent and positive interactions with people who could provide mentoring and support. For them, it was a renewal of a relationship with a member of their extended family that provided that support.

### Making Meaning of Experiences

Finally, there is growing evidence that the cognitive and affective processing of experience is important to reducing the risk and strengthening self-esteem and relationships (Rutter, 1999). Children need a coherent, meaningful story that ties the events of their lives together, connects them with their families and support systems, and gives meaning to their experiences. Narrative therapy (Cattanach, 2008; Freeman, Epston, & Lobovits, 1997) provides play therapists with an outline of how to help children and their families develop stories about themselves and their families that are not problem-saturated but strengths-based.

Michael, the bright but sad 10-year-old failing classes and becoming socially withdrawn, came for play therapy sessions for a number of months. His family history included spending most of his 10 years with very limited contact with his father, who was in and out of his life. He lived with his mother, who had a series of relationships over the 10 years; several of the partners had taken interest in Michael and then left when the relationship with his mother ended. He played out in session this theme of gaining and losing relationships in any number of ways, with people figures searching for a lost person and with stuffed animals searching for lost babies. Over time, in play sessions, in sessions with his mother, and with consultations with the school, Michael began a process of healing from these multiple griefs. He became more socially outgoing, his school performance improved, and he began a martial arts program. He became a voracious reader and writer, and sometimes he brought samples of stories he wrote, both for school and for his own enjoyment.

Building on this newly discovered interest in writing, and wanting to help Michael sustain his progress, the therapist asked him one day, "Michael, if you were to write a story about experiences in this play therapy room, and the changes you have made in your life, what would you write about?" He thought a bit, then brightened, and said, "I would write the Lost and Found Story!" The theme that had been a metaphor for his pain, and the relief from his pain, had stayed with him these many months. It took on new meaning as he plunged into the project of writing the story. It became the focus of discussion in several sessions and in numerous conversations with his mother at home for several weeks. In his own words, in his own way, he had made some sense of his experience; his story expressed and respected his pain, honored his efforts, and pointed to a future. As the narrative therapists point out, stories are indeed transformational.

## RESILIENCE AND PLAY THERAPY BEYOND THE PLAY THERAPY ROOM

Play therapy sessions provide a safe and creative place for children and their families to develop and enhance qualities of resiliency. Rutter's resiliency model can provide a practical framework of guidelines for play therapists to integrate the powers of play into their work with children and their families. The resiliency research also points therapists to issues of family, community, and culture that can contribute to developing resilience in children (Buckley, Thorngren, & Kleist, 1997; Waller, 2001). In an extensive review of promising practices in child mental health (Simpson, Jivanjee, Koroloff, Doerfler, & García, 2001), four major qualities of successful child mental health services were identified, and all four play a role in the provision of play therapy: coordinated transdisciplinary treatment, focus on the developmental needs of the child, encouragement of family participation in care, and empowerment of families through strengths and resilience. These "beyond the session" factors suggest that play therapists must expand their understanding of therapeutic processes and their therapeutic role to include a role in working with families, consulting with key members of the child's support system, and advocating regarding social problems that contribute to the societal sources of risk. As Masten (2001) stated, "If major threats to children are those adversities that undermine basic protective systems for development, it follows that efforts to promote competence and resilience in children at risk should focus on strategies that protect or restore the efficacy of these basic systems" (p. 235).

## REFERENCES

Bratton, S., & Ray, D. (2000). What the research shows about play therapy. *International Journal of Play Therapy, 9*, 47–88.

Brooks, R. B. (1994a). Children at risk: Fostering resilience and hope. *American Journal of Orthopsychiatry, 64*, 545–553.

Brooks, R. B. (1994b). Diagnostic issues and therapeutic interventions for children at risk. *American Journal of Orthopsychiatry, 64*, 508–509.

Buckley, M. R., Thorngren, J. M., & Kleist, D. M. (1997). Family resiliency: A neglected family construct. *The Family Journal: Counseling and Therapy for Couples and Families, 5*, 241–246.

Cattanach, A. (2008). *Narrative approaches in play with children*. London: Jessica Kingsley.

Crenshaw, D. A. (2006). *Evocative strategies in child and adolescent psychotherapy*. Lanham, MD: Jason Aronson.

Crenshaw, D. A. (2008). *Therapeutic engagement of children and adolescents: Play, symbol, drawing, and storytelling strategies*. Lanham, MD: Jason Aronson.

Freeman, J., Epston, D., & Lobovits, D. (1997). *Playful approaches to serious problems: Narrative therapy with children and their families*. New York: W. W. Norton.

Garbarino, J. (1994). *Raising children in a socially toxic environment*. San Francisco: Jossey-Bass.

Gil, E. (1994). *Play in family therapy*. New York: Guilford Press.

Gil, E. (2006). *Helping abused and traumatized children: Integrating directive and non-directive approaches*. New York: Guilford Press.

Gil, E., & Sobol, B. (2000). Engaging families in therapeutic play. In C. E. Bailey (Ed.), *Children in therapy: Using the family as a resource* (pp. 314–283). New York: W. W. Norton.

Goldstein, S., & Brooks, R. B. (Eds.). (2006). *Handbook of resilience in children*. New York: Springer Science.

Guerney, L. (1991). Parents as partners in treating behavior problems in early childhood settings. *Topics in Early Childhood (Special Ed.), 11*, 74–90.

Guerney, L. (1997). Filial therapy. In K. J. O'Connor & E. M. Braverman (Eds.), *Play therapy theory and practice: A comparative presentation* (pp.130–159). New York: John Wiley.

Jernberg, A., & Booth, P. (1999). *Theraplay* (2nd ed.). San Francisco: Jossey-Bass.

Johnson, A. C. (1995). Resiliency mechanisms in culturally diverse families. *The Family Journal: Counseling and Therapy for Couples and Families, 3*, 316–324.

Knell, S. (1993). *Cognitive-behavioral play therapy*. Northvale, NJ: Jason Aronson.

Kottman, T. (2002). *Partners in play: Adlerian play therapy* (2nd ed.). Alexandria, VA: American Counseling Association.

Landreth, G. L. (2002). *Play therapy: The art of relationship* (2nd ed.). Philadelphia: Taylor & Francis.

Landreth, G. L., & Bratton, S. C. (2006a). *Child Parent Relationship Therapy (CPRT): A 10-session filial therapy model*. New York: Routledge.

Landreth, G. L., & Bratton, S. C. (2006b). *Child Parent Relationship Therapy (CPRT): Treatment manual*. New York: Routledge.

LeBlanc, M., & Ritchie, M. (2001). A meta-analysis of play therapy outcomes. *Counseling Psychology Quarterly, 14*, 149–163.

Masten, A. (2001). Ordinary magic: Resilience processes in development. *American Psychologist, 56*, 227–238.

Oaklander, V. (1992). *Windows to our children: A Gestalt therapy approach to children and adolescents*. Highland, NY: Gestalt Journal Press.

O'Connor, K. J. (2000). *Play therapy primer* (2nd ed.). New York: John Wiley.

Perry, B. D. (2006). The Neurosequential Model of Therapeutics: Applying principles of neuroscience to clinical work with traumatized and maltreated children. In N. B. Webb (Ed.), *Working with traumatized youth in child welfare* (pp. 27–52). New York: Guilford Press.

Perry, B. D., & Hanbrick, E. P. (2008). The neurosequential model of therapeutics. *Reclaiming Children and Youth, 17*, 38–43.

Quinton, D., & Rutter, M. (1988). *Parenting breakdown: The making and breaking of inter-generational links*. Aldershot, UK: Avebury.

Ray, D., Bratton, S., Rhine, T., & Jones, L. (2001). The effectiveness of play therapy: Responding to the critics. *International Journal of Play Therapy, 10*, 85–108.

Rutter, M. (1971). Parent-child separation: Psychological effects on the children. *Journal of Child Psychology and Psychiatry, 12*, 233–260.

Rutter, M. E. (1987). Psychosocial resilience and protective mechanisms. *American Journal of Orthopsychiatry, 57*, 316–331.

Rutter, M. E. (1993). Resilience: Some conceptual considerations. *Journal of Adolescent Health, 14,* 626–631.

Rutter, M. E. (1999). Resilience concepts and findings: Implications for family therapy. *Journal of Family Therapy, 21,* 119–144.

Rutter, M. E. (2007). Resilience, competence, and coping. *Child Abuse & Neglect, 31,* 205–209.

Rutter, M. E., & Rutter, M. (1993). *Developing minds: Challenge and continuity across the lifespan.* New York: Basic Books.

Schaefer, C. E. (1993). *The therapeutic powers of play.* Northvale, NJ: Jason Aronson.

Schaefer, C. E., & Carey, L. J. (Eds.). (1994). *Family play therapy.* Northvale, NJ: Jason Aronson.

Schaefer, C. E., & Kaduson, H. G. (Eds.). (2006). *Contemporary play therapy: Theory, research, and practice.* New York: Guilford Press.

Seymour, J. W., & Erdman, P. (1996). Family play therapy using a resilience model. *International Journal of Play Therapy, 5,* 19–30.

Shapiro, J. P., & Friedman, D. (1996, November 11). Invincible kids. *U.S. News & World Report, 121*(19), 62–71.

Simpson, J., Jivanjee, P., Koroloff, N., Doerfler, A., & García, M. (2001). *Systems of care: Promising practices in children's mental health, 2001 series* (Vol. 3). Washington, DC: Center for Effective Collaboration and Practice, American Institutes for Research.

Smokowski, P. R. (1998). Prevention and intervention strategies for promoting resilience in disadvantaged children. *Social Service Review, 72,* 337–364.

Terr, L. (1990). *Too scared to cry.* New York: Basic Books.

VanFleet, R. (1994a). *Filial therapy: Strengthening parent-child relationships.* Sarasota, FL: Professional Resource Exchange.

VanFleet, R. (1994b). *Filial therapy: Strengthening parent-child relationships through play.* Sarasota, FL: Professional Resource Press.

VanFleet, R. (2000). *A parent's handbook of filial therapy: Building strong families with play.* Boiling Springs, PA: Play Therapy Press.

VanFleet, R., & Guerney, L. (Eds.). (2003). *A casebook of filial therapy.* Boiling Springs, PA: The Family Enhancement and Play Therapy Center.

Waller, M. A. (2001). Resilience in ecosystemic context: Evolution of the concept. *American Journal of Orthopsychiatry, 71,* 290–297.

Walsh, F. (2002). A family resilience framework: Innovative practice application. *Family Relations, 51,* 130–137.

Walsh, F. (2003). Family resilience: Strengths forged through adversity. In F. Walsh (Ed.), *Normal family process: Growing diversity and complexity* (pp. 399–423). New York: Guilford Press.

Webb, N. B. (Ed.). (1999). *Play therapy with children in crisis: Individual, group, and family treatment* (2nd ed.). New York: Guilford Press

Wright, M. O., & Masten, A. S. (2006). Resilience processes in development. In S. Goldstein & R. B. Brooks (Eds.), *Handbook of resilience in children* (pp. 17–38). New York: Springer.

# 6

# A Strengths-Based Approach to Dynamically Oriented Child Therapy

*Steven Tuber*

I begin this chapter with the single most formative experience of my career as a psychologist. It embodies the essence of a strengths-based approach to diagnosis and hence to treatment, as we cannot begin to know how to be of help to anyone before we attempt to fully understand them. I call it the "Patty Story." I tell it every year as the very first statement I make to my first-year graduate students in the doctoral program in clinical psychology at the City College of New York. I always want to give it the "primacy effect" it deserves. I have been told numerous times over the years that it remains the most salient story many of these graduate students take away from their graduate training. Here's the story.

I was working in a community mental health center near the start of my career. One of my roles was to serve as a liaison with our local foster care agency regarding children placed in their care. I was asked to assess a five-year-old girl. Her mother had been institutionalized off and on for major depression throughout her only child's life, beginning when "Patty" was nine months old. Patty's mom was a single mom in her mid-20s, with enormous struggles financially as well. She was about to be released again from the hospital and the question was whether Patty was robust and healthy enough to once again tolerate a transition from her stable foster care situation to living alone with her mom. To make matters more difficult, Patty had been diagnosed as an infant with a physiological delay such that a sizable percentage of her myelin sheath development surrounding many of her nerve endings in her skin was insufficient, making even the slightest of maternal caresses a lesson in pain for Patty. Without ever even seeing Patty or her mom, I just "knew" this child must be quite disturbed! After all, she had a significantly limited and troubled mom, a socioeconomic status that put her at equally great risk and limitation and a neurophysiological early status that would have subsumed most of the supremely important first year of her life within a shroud of physical as well as emotional pain. So despite a single, stable foster care family that treated her with kindness off and on during her first five years, this child had "no chance" of being a healthy child, or so I thought.

So imagine my surprise when I met Patty in consultation. She was everything I thought she couldn't be. She was warm, curious, engaging but appropriately bounded and not indiscriminate in any of these characteristics. She could play symbolically and with gusto and the themes of her play were utterly age and developmentally vital. She spoke with pleasure of her mom's imminent return, yet could acknowledge both sadness and even a bit of anger at her frequent disappearances. Not believing what I was experiencing, I clung to my belief in psychopathological reductionism—this girl had to be more disturbed that she appeared, it must be some sort of "false self" (Tuber, 2008) façade she was presenting, and hiding beneath this façade was the pathology that "had" to be there. I asked to see her again and was made even more befuddled by our second session, in which she was every bit as alive and healthy as in the first, but with an even warmer connection to the "feelings doctor" she had come to see again!

I sheepishly called the foster care agency, told my contact there what I had observed and asked to meet with Patty's mother and asked to read Patty's mom's psychiatric record. I had told myself that this mom had to have been misdiagnosed; it was the "only" thing I could think of to solve this riddle of a healthy child coming from such a "pathological" place. Yet mom's psychiatric history was nearly the size of the Manhattan Yellow Pages; surely so troubled a woman could not be an adequate parent!

Patty's mom entered my office looking like a caricature of a depressed person. She looked haggard, almost twice her chronological age, with hunched shoulders, an almost shuffling gait and a look of resignation I found painful to witness. There was no way such a woman, however well-intentioned, could have produced such a delightful child! We began speaking and I soon asked her about Patty and especially about Patty's first year of life. Although she lightened considerably at the mention of Patty's name, a consideration of Patty's first months led her to lose eye contact and, head downcast, she told me of how guilty she felt about that time, how she had been so depressed just after Patty was born and felt miserably about the mother she had been to her. I asked her to paint me a scene of exactly what she had done with Patty, pushing her to help me get a glimpse of the phenomenological or "actual experience" (Escalona, 1969) of Patty at that time. She spoke of how she barely had the energy to move in those early weeks and months but would lie sadly on the couch in her small apartment. She had one of those baby seats that could prop the infant in an almost vertical position and kept Patty loosely swaddled in this chair right next to her on the couch. She noted that she had one real gift—she had a beautiful singing voice so she remembered keeping Patty right next to her, inches away, and sang to her off and on all day. She was crying softly as she said this and my eyes were wet with tears as well. After several quiet moments, I finally said to her that not only was she understandably moved by that meaningful time in her baby's life, but that she had actually given her baby exactly what she needed—she couldn't have done a better job! For given Patty's neurophysiologic delays, a more typically affectionate parent would have left Patty in pain with each touch, while what Patty received from her mom was loving, soothing, reliable, auditory and visual contact, the exact two senses Patty could experience with pain-free delight.

No wonder Patty was so much healthier than I had "deduced"—her first year phenomenology was of an attuned, available, "good enough" (Winnicott, 1971) mother helping her to create an experience of self and other that was also "good enough." The model of pathology I was trained in: disturbed, single mother + physiologically delayed child = child pathology had been overruled by a new equation: devoted, willing, mother + infant receiving attuned care = healthy internalized representations of self and other in a vitally developing child.

It's clear to me that despite being blessed with a number of great teachers in my own training, Patty and her mom were my greatest teachers. I have tried ever since, with every child and adult I treat, to keep Patty in mind and to strive to obtain as holistic and attuned appraisal of each person who enters my office as I can, knowing that their strengths often lie just below a wellspring of pathology that may or may not be relevant to their ongoing struggles. If life is, as Ibsen noted, "to do battle with trolls," it is essential to know what strengths our patients bring to this battle if we are to be of any use to them.

With this "prologue" in mind, I'd like to first say a word or two about the nature of in-depth, psychodynamically oriented play therapy in the context of a strengths-based approach to treatment. Such an approach can easily stir up (and occasionally warrant) antagonisms: its lack of a "manual" or systemized approach invites a wallowing in pathology, it is said; it presents no time frame for termination, inviting a type of witch hunt for a never-ending series of symptoms or difficulties; it ignores the need for a child/family to work things out on their own, etc. I cannot refute any of these claims, nor would I ever want to preclude them from an open discussion as to the merits of psychotherapy in general or psychodynamically oriented treatment in particular. I do want to affirm the possibility that all the obverse claims about this approach can be equally true. An indefinite-term, in-depth treatment of a child lends enormous respect to the child's ability to heal; it gives real, profound affirmation of how damaging earlier suffering can be and therefore equal weight to serving as a catalyst in the battle against such psychic pain and it constantly enlists the aid of the child's ego resources as the very basis for its utility and process.

With this "controversy" in mind and with a focus on the affirmation and utilization of the child's ego resources as the cornerstone of in-depth therapy, I would like to present three vignettes, all part of the same play session with a six-year-old girl. The girl, I'll call her Sally, had two huge strikes against her, much as Patty did. In Sally's case, profound marital conflict in Sally's second and third years of life led to many scenes of threatened and actual physical abuse between her parents. This "strike" was paired with significant language processing delays on Sally's part, making the process of learning to read and write a nightmare. Sally was becoming increasingly withdrawn and restless at school, culminating in a diagnosis of Attention Deficit Disorder with Hyperactivity. She had had a psychiatric consultation just before I began treating her, with a decision made to defer medication for six months to see how psychotherapy might affect her functioning. I began seeing Sally twice weekly in play therapy. She was a moving, poignant person, with a capacity for bravery and a willingness to take on difficult feelings that I have always found to be worthy of my full respect.

All three vignettes come from her 24th session with me. The first is a strikingly courageous struggle with her experience of witnessed aggression between her parents.

("S" is Sally, "T" is Tuber)

*S*: Listen to this! Drawing the elephant, drawing the elephant, presenting the elephant, the famous one and only elephant in the world. There's only one elephant in the universe. Presenting the elephant. Presenting the elephant. Look at the elephant, look at the elephant. Elephants marching. Elephant, elephant, elephant, elephant. Come with me on a marching band. Elephant, elephant, who are you? Get out of this town (scolding tone). I hate elephants! Who are you? Get out!

*T*: One minute the elephants are coming and are so special, the next minute they're gotten rid of like they're nothing!

*S*: This woman (picks up a doll figure) is yelling at them.

*S*: Get out of town!

*T*: Get out of town you elephants!

*S*: This old crabby lady is yelling at them: "Get out of town!" The elephants are here to stay! No, get those elephants out of town. I hate elephants, get them out! Get them out! I hate elephants!

*T*: Why does that lady now hate those elephants so much?

*S*: Because when she was four years old, one stepped on her.

*T*: Oh my goodness, now I understand! So she's been scared and mad at elephants ever since she was four years old; such a long time to be scared and mad!

*S*: That's why she's a crabby woman.

(She takes the doll figure and pushes it toward me in a mock attack.)

*S*: Who said I was crabby?

*T*: Now she's accusing me of being mean but I didn't say it.

*S*: It wasn't me. I didn't say something crazy about myself! So just get those elephants out of this town. I order you to!

*T*: She's so angry she wants everyone to listen to her orders!

*S*: What's that you say (in crabby voice)?

*T*: I said you're angry at those elephants because of what they did to you when you were a little girl.

*S*: (Softer voice) Those were different elephants that did that.

*T*: Then why do you want to get rid of these elephants?

*T*: One moment the elephants could be so kind and the next moment so wild!

*S*: Yes (talking as the doll) I'm afraid they'll do that to me now! Oh, help, help! One's about to step on me! (She moves the picture of the elephant toward her play figure in an attacking way.)

(I move her figure out of the way at the last moment.)

*T*: You're right lady. You're afraid that things that happened to you when you were little will come back and scare you and make you feel bad and worried forever and ever.

*S*: Oh, beware the elephants! That lady was very grumpy to the elephants.

*T*: I understand they were very grumpy to her when she was little.

*S*: By accident! She didn't know the elephants couldn't see her because she was so small.

*T*: I think when she was so little she didn't understand it was an accident. She thought they were doing something mean on purpose.

*S*: So she turned into a crabby old lady when she grew up. That's why you have to understand feelings!

*T*: It's true.

*S*: You'll turn into a crabby lady if you don't.

*T*: Or sometimes you can turn into a scared and sad one too, with crabby feelings on the outside but sad ones on the inside.

*S*: I'm going to draw again now. (She turns to her drawing and covers her work.)

*T*: OK, I'll close my eyes.

*S*: Wait, don't look. I'm drawing the grass and something. Can you turn the other way? You can keep your eyes open, just turn the other way.

(I turn my chair; she sings to herself and draws with pleasure.)

There are many ways to enter into a discussion about this moment in a therapy. For the purposes of the present chapter, I want to focus on this girl's bravery. The essence of bravery for me is to be willing to let one's self enter a psychological arena where you have no real way of knowing how to proceed and where it will lead. She begins this vignette identifying with the aggressor, proclaiming the power and uniqueness of this massive creature. It would have been "easy" and understandable if she remained content with this identification. Quickly, however, she adds another character that has the temerity to rail against this hateful beast. She demands the ouster of the elephant despite how small and frail she is in comparison. This is brave enough, yet she immediately responds to my question about why this woman is so full of hate. She relates it back to her childhood and the feelings of being small, inconsequential, and thus at the mercy of being obliterated. While in the character of the "crabby" woman, she tries to enlist my aid in getting rid of the elephant, then movingly notes how there seems to be two kinds of elephants, a strikingly accurate picture of her early actual experience with two well-meaning but unpredictably volatile parents. When the elephant turns on her in the play, we enact a rescue scene that allows her to reflect on her past experience with a remarkably adept degree of reflective functioning ("that's why you have to understand feelings") and an awareness of outcome ("you'll turn into a crabby lady if you don't") that would make any scholar of mentalizing or reflective capabilities proud (Fonagy et al., 2002)! I am on another level struck by the creativity of her shifting identifications. This child, despite many painful early experiences, had a true capacity for play. As I have discussed elsewhere (Tuber, 2008), play "provides the most original means for the child to expand and process reality" (p. 4). The attainment of the capacity to play is not a given; it is a hard-won developmental achievement easily lost if reality is traumatizing. Sally's originality and creativity (in this vignette alone, she can shift her voice from elephant to old woman to child and simultaneously use a drawing and a doll figure to connote a true-to-life drama) depict a capacity to play at a very high level. This capacity, in turn, implies several major psychological attainments: the capacity to be alone in the presence of another; the ability to create a third, "intermediate" space not solely internal or external wherein the drama is presented; the attainment of a "True Self" in which authenticity predominates and the means to "use" others to further develop this sense of aliveness (Tuber, 2008, p. 4). For Sally to be this advanced despite a prolonged period of parental discord speaks directly to her (and her parents') courage and resilience.

The second vignette with Sally focuses on her phenomenological experience of her difficulties in understanding written language. It is important to contrast her actual experience (Escalona, 1969) with her psychiatric diagnosis of ADHD. In earlier writings, I have discussed many of the limitations of such a deficit-based, symptom-focused diagnostic approach (Tuber et al., 2007; Harris et al., 2006). I have echoed the work of Gilmore (2000, 2002) and Stormont (2001), among many others, who emphasize that ADHD has to be looked at in the context of the multidimensional interplay between developmental, intrapsychic, constitutional, and environmental factors. In Sally's case, what could be easily missed in the context of her "spacey," restless school behavior was the enormous confusion experienced in the context of learning how to link word sounds with letters as symbols. The following first portion of the vignette speaks vividly to her letting me know directly how bewildered her experience was in this arena:

*S*: I know how to make a picture—do you have some stencils or anything—I need to draw with a stencil.

(She begins to draw her name in tiny letters at the top of her page.)

*S*: Can you write your name in the tiny little space at the top?

*T*: You want it to be very, very small?

*S*: Is that really small?

*T*: Wow! That is very small.

*S*: I don't think people can read my name. (Then points to my name on my paper.)

*S*: On the top of your paper!

*T*: Oh, mine's not on the very top.

*S*: Is mine? (We look at her paper, she seems satisfied.)

*S*: Can you write in script?

*T*: It's not an easy thing to learn at first.

*S*: (After watching me sign my name) You're not writing anything!

*T*: It seems weird to you but that's my name in script and that's my name in print.

*S*: (She seems confused.) How do you spell: ah, ah eeek!? (giggles)

*T*: I have no idea—those sounds feel so confusing!

*S*: How do you spell: wah!?

*T*: How do you spell wah? Seems like you're coming up with sounds to spell, it's so hard to spell sounds, it makes me feel dumb.

*S*: Sound it out (in scolding tone): wah-ah-ah-eeek! (giggles)

*T*: What could possibly spell a wah-ah-ah-eek sound?

*S*: Wah eek, eeee, wah ah eeek!

*T*: Trying to sound out the terrible wah-ah-eek!

*S*: Mah, oooh, oooh. (She begins writing letters on the page that roughly conform to the sounds she made.)

*T*: You're spelling out all kinds of special sounds.

*S*: Rrrggg! Try that one! Sound out that! Sound out running. How do you sound out running? Do you think it's hard to sound out running? It's easy! Let me sound out running. (She runs around saying the cat running, cat running.)

*T*: You're not only sounding it out—it feels better to act it out!

*S*: Yes!

*T*: You're sounding it out and running at the same time.

*S*: Is this acting it? (She "turns into" a statue.)

*T*: Acting like a statue, a laughing statue!

*S*: Is this acting too? (She juggles a pencil.)

*T*: Acting like a pencil juggler! (She giggles.)

*S*: Is this acting too? (She spins around on my ottoman while on her belly, yelling move! Move!) (I have no idea what she's up to.)

*T*: This feels like you're mind is spinning from one idea to the next, it's so hard to know what you're feeling or thinking now.

(S nods her head, stops spinning and goes back to her drawing.)

It is striking to follow the progression of these two minutes of a treatment session. She begins by wanting a stencil, a device to make sure she doesn't make a mistake. When this is not available, she bravely begins writing one of the very few things she can write, her name, and wants confirmation that she can at least write it in as small a print as possible, although she doubts whether its "readable." She asks me to write in script and when I do so, it exacerbates her limitations and confusions. She then immediately turns the table on me and uses the rest of the vignette to present a series of nonsense sounds that mirror her experience of how random and chaotic the learning to read process has been for her. It's also striking how the very act of trying to sound out words is so dysregulating for her that she launches into a running external enactment of her inner experience of being out of control. In an earlier paper, my colleagues and I wrote about this experience in the following way:

> With low tolerance for intense affect and anxiety, children with ADHD can become easily dysregulated by unexpected changes in their environment and by the dynamic quality inherent in social exchanges. They may then appear . . . hyper-excitable and anxious. (Harris et al., 2006, p. 500)

This exemplifies Sally at that moment in the session.

Later in the same session, Sally addresses her difficulties in the use of written language in a dramatically different fashion. She had asked me to draw an elephant and we had had many exchanges in the past where my poor ability to draw has been used by Sally as a source of comfort, identification, and/or an avenue to express how cruel others had been to her about her deficiencies. This is the third vignette:

> (She looks at my drawing.)
>
> *S*: Cool, that looks like a "v."
>
> *T*: That looks like a "v" for a tail?
>
> *S*: I thought pigs had curly tails, not tails that look like "v's."
>
> *T*: My elephant's tail also doesn't seem good enough.
>
> *S*: An elephant (with mock indignation)? I thought it was a pig!
>
> *T*: You asked me to draw an elephant and instead it looks like a pig?
>
> *S*: You're not a pig.
>
> *T*: I'm glad you don't think I'm a pig! (S giggles.)
>
> *S*: But you smell like one!
>
> *T*: Ooof!
>
> *S*: Do you know what pigs smell like? . . . What's your favorite food?
>
> *T*: What's my . . . pigs smell like my favorite food?!
>
> *S*: (giggles) What's your favorite food?
>
> *T*: Suddenly you're making my favorite food very stinky!
>
> (S giggles.)
>
> *S*: Is that your favorite food (pointing to drawing)? No.
>
> *T*: First you turn my elephant into a smelly animal and then you turn my favorite food into a smelly, stinky one. (S giggles.)
>
> *S*: I have an idea.

*T*: OK

*S*: Can you do this? (She begins to play at knotting up her fingers.)

*T*: I don't think so.

*S*: Do it!

*T*: I'll try, but I don't think I can.

*S*: Can you do this? I don't think I can. I don't think I can. I don't think I can (in a mocking, dismissing tone).

*T*: I know one thing you are doing.

*S*: What?

*T*: You can copy me and make fun of me when I seem weak or clumsy.

*S*: I know one thing I can't do.

*T*: What's that?

(S gestures, acting as if she can't speak.)

*T*: Talk?

(S gestures again that she lost her voice.)

*T*: Something's happened between us and you can't speak!

*S*: Only ask me yes or no questions—wait a minute, can I use this for something?

(She begins to cut up small pieces of paper from a larger piece).

*T*: I wonder what could make her voice go away.

*S*: (whispers) Shh! Only ask me yes or no questions.

(I see that she has written the words yes and no on two separate pieces of paper.)

*T*: I think I understand. You want my words but your answers are for me to see but not hear. You want me to ask you more questions?

(She picks up both the yes and no papers.)

*T*: No, yes. You're not sure. A little bit no and a little bit yes.

(S takes a third scrap of paper and writes "yes and no" on it.)

*T*: Ahh. Sometimes you have both yes and no feelings to the same question.

(S nods and whispers yes and no to herself.)

*T*: Only yes or no questions, I should only ask questions that have yes or no for an answer?

*S*: (whispers) Questions that have yes or no answers, nothing else! If you get a no, it's a question I don't like.

*T*: I see.

*S*: And I don't have to answer it. And I don't want to answer it.

*T*: I see. If I ask a question you don't like, you're just going to put up the no and if it's a question that you like, you'll say yes?

*S*: I'll say yes and I'll answer the question!

*T*: Sometimes I ask questions that you don't like. Yes or no?

(S shows me the "yes" piece of paper.)

*T*: Sometimes I ask you questions that make you angry at me.

(S shows me the "yes" paper.)

*T*: Sometimes I ask you questions and you don't know the answers to them and that makes you feel small and weak.

(S shows me the "yes" paper.)

*T*: And sometimes it's hard for you to understand why I would ask you those kinds of questions.

(S shows me the "yes and no" paper.)

*T*: Yes and no. You can understand some of it but not all of it. Sometimes you understand that I ask you questions because I want us to both understand what you're feeling.

(S shows me the "yes" paper.)

*T*: And sometimes it just doesn't make any sense at all why I ask you a question.

(S whispers, "Sometimes.")

*T*: Sometimes yes and sometimes no?

*S*: That's true.

*T*: You could use a "sometimes" card.

*S*: I do need a "sometimes" card. How do you spell sometimes?

*T*: It's a long word. (I spell it out for her while she writes it on another scrap of paper.)

*S*: Sometimes.

*S*: How do you spell, "I don't know"? (I spell it as she writes it on a fifth scrap of paper.)

*T*: Now you have five cards that can answer so many things: "Yes," "no," "yes and no," "sometimes," and "I don't know." We should keep these cards for next time so that if I have any questions. . . .

*S*: Oh, don't have us stop!

*T*: You don't want us to stop; you want me to ask lots more questions?

(S whispers, "a little more.")

*T*: I think we have time for two more questions.

*S*: All right.

*T*: Ok.

*S*: Hurry up!

*T*: Sometimes you have many different feelings when you come to see me.

(S first shows the "sometimes" card, then the "I don't know" card.)

*T*: You don't know if you know the answer to that one. And one more question. Sometimes it's very hard for you to say goodbye and have to wait until the next time we meet.

(S shows me the "yes" card.)

*S*: I like these cards. (She laughs warmly and begins to spell out phonetically the word "certainly" and writes it on another scrap of paper.)

*T*: Certainly. Certainly I know it's hard to wait but I will see you next time and we do have to stop for today.

(I begin to gather the papers and place them in her folder that is nearby. She gets up to leave.)

*S*: When is the next time?

*T*: Oh, Thursday at our regular time, two days from now.

(She has written several question marks on another piece of paper after she had asked me when the next time to meet was.)

*T*: You have good question marks and good questions too.

(She nods and leaves the room easily.)

She begins this stretch of the session by at first humorously but then more belligerently being verbally hostile. At first I'm able to engage and acknowledge her aggression, being comfortable with her making me "smelly." Regrettably, something about her mocking my words gets under my skin and I "retaliate" by telling her she was making fun of me. My inability to withstand this form of my patient's "hate" reminds me of D. W. Winnicott's warning in working deeply with patients that the therapist, "must be prepared to bear strain without expecting the patient to know anything about what he is doing, perhaps over a long period of time. To do this he must be easily aware of his own fear and hate" (Winnicott, 1949, p. 198). So what does Sally do in the face of my retaliation? She turns the tables beautifully by saying she's lost her voice! "Turning lemons into lemonade," she creatively takes her great difficulties with the written word (and with me at that moment) and converts her interactions with me into a series of written "flash cards" that convey enormous meaning through the very modality she more typically associates with incompetence and inadequacy. She does this, moreover, exactly at a moment when I am least with her, again revealing an enormous faith in her True Self, even when I am not being attuned enough to her needs. Her courageous capacity to play in this difficult moment readily confirms Erikson's comment that "man is perfectly human only when he plays" (Haworth, 1964, p. 4). I was also struck by how her production of the cards gradually expanded from two to four to six by the end of the session, serving as a prototype for exactly the kind of generalization and development we most hope for from our patients. Her ability to take her weakness and turn it into an adaptive, highly communicative strength is, to my mind, the epitome of a demonstration of the power to self-repair. By bearing witness to such creative processes in our patients, we cannot help but develop a deeper appreciation for the notion of a strengths-based approach, especially in the context of an in-depth treatment of indeterminate length.

## REFERENCES

Erikson, E. (1964). Toys and reasons. In M. Haworth (Ed.) *Child psychotherapy* (pp. 3–10). New York: Basic Books.

Escalona, S. (1969). *The roots of individuality*. Chicago: Aldine.

Fonagy, P., Gergely, G., Jurist, E., & Target, M. (2002). *Affect regulation, mentalization and the development of the self*. New York: Other Press.

Gilmore, K. (2000). A psychoanalytic perspective on Attentional-Deficit/Hyperactivity Disorder. *Journal of the American Psychiatric Association, 48*(4), 1259–1293.

Gilmore, K. (2002). Diagnosis, dynamics and development: Considerations in the psychoanalytic assessment of children with ADHD. *Psychoanalytic Inquiry, 22*(3), 372–390.

Harris, B., Reynoso, J., Meehan, K., Ueng-McHale, J., & Tuber, S. (2006). A child with ADHD: Convergences of Rorschach data and case material. *Journal of Infant, Child and Adolescent Psychotherapy, 5*(4), 499–517.

Haworth, M. (1964). *Child psychotherapy: practice and theory*. New York: Basic Books.

Stormont, M. (2001). Social outcomes of children with ADHD: Contributing factors and implications for practice. *Psychology in the Schools, 38*(6), 521–531.

Tuber, S. (2008). *Attachment, play and authenticity: A Winnicott primer*. Lanham, MD: Jason Aronson.

Tuber, S., Harris, B., Meehan, K., Reynoso, J., & Ueng-McHale, J. (2007). Rorschach configurations of children with ADHD. In S. Smith & L. Handler (Eds.), *The*

*Clinical assessment of children and adolescents* (pp. 451–468). Mahwah, NJ: Lawrence Erlbaum.

Winnicott, D. W. (1949). Hate in the countertransference. In *Through pediatrics to psychoanalysis* (pp. 194–203). New York: Basic Books.

Winnicott, D. W. (1971). *Playing and reality*. London: Tavistock Publications.

# 7

# Overcoming All Odds: Helping Young Men Find Their Strengths

*Gregory Barker*

As he took the stage with his family on election night, the crowd rose in unison in Grant Park in Chicago. Many will never forget that image of the first African American striding to the podium to deliver his presidential acceptance speech before 250,000 joyful and tearful souls. Barack Obama had just been elected the 44th president of the United States. Older members of the crowd uniformly expressed their disbelief: "I never thought I would ever see in my lifetime a black man elected to be president of the United States."

Despite what appeared to be overwhelming odds when he announced his candidacy for president 21 months earlier, Barack Obama had ascended to the most powerful position in the world. Many of the elders in the crowd had witnessed the aftermath of the assassination of Martin Luther King on their grainy black and white television sets in 1968. They had seen news clips of Bull Connor and his police attack dogs in Birmingham, Governor George Wallace blocking the schoolhouse door to desegregation at the University of Alabama, Rosa Parks's refusal to be seated in the rear of the bus, the Watts Riots, and civil rights marches on Washington in the late 1960s. It's no wonder they couldn't conceive of Obama's ascent to power that night, a man who represented a culture and a race that had been oppressed since the origins of North American slavery in 1619.

As biographers write of Obama's life, the term "resilience" will emerge as a predominant characteristic that helped carry him to a position of prominence on the world stage. Pundits will offer their opinions about how his sense of determination shaped his personality. They will reread and analyze Obama's books *Dreams from My Father* and *The Audacity of Hope* in order to gain insight into the part of his personality that provided him with a venue for overcoming all odds. Obama clarifies in his autobiographical works the many struggles and obstacles facing a young man of mixed race without a father. In many ways, Obama's overall life serves as a symbol of the successful negotiation of cultural, racial, and gender dilemmas that young men confront on their path to adulthood. Obama's story symbolizes resilience at its best.

## CHALLENGES IN COUNSELING WITH YOUNG MEN

During the past 15 years, there has been a dramatic shift in the interest regarding the health of young men in American culture. Research literature has begun to attest to the distinct and separate issues facing boys as they adjust to difficulties during childhood and adolescence. The differences in the challenges between girls and boys are difficult to dispute. The facts and statistics are convincing.

- One thousand nine hundred fifteen males under the age of 20 were murdered in 2005 (U.S. Department of Justice, Federal Bureau of Investigation, 2006).
- Boys commit suicide more frequently than girls. In 2001, 86 percent of all youth suicides were committed by boys (Centers for Disease Control and Prevention, 2007).
- Sixteen percent of men report that they were the victims of child abuse (Baker & King, 2004).
- Young men drop out of high school at higher rates than women by age 19. Twenty-four percent of boys fail to graduate; the figure for girls is 17 percent.
- Seventy-four percent of all delinquency offenses are committed by boys (U.S. Census Bureau, 2007).
- The suicide rate among gay boys accounts for about 30 percent of all adolescent suicides (Borowsky, Ireland, & Resnick, 2001).
- Between 1967 and 2000, the proportion of 18- to 24-year-old female high school graduates that were enrolled in college increased by 20.5 percent. For men of the same age, the number enrolled in college decreased by 3.8 percent (U.S. Census Bureau).
- Males represent a shrinking share of the bachelor's degrees in every major field of study (National Center for Education Statistics).
- In K–12 education, boys are more likely to be diagnosed with special education needs than girls. Among high school students, 73 percent of those with learning disabilities and 76 percent of those who were labeled "emotionally disturbed" are boys (U.S. Department of Education).

Over the past 30 years, I have counseled and worked with boys who are described as "high-risk" youth in residential centers, school settings, hospitals, and private practice. It is my impression that a number of intersecting biological and social factors account for many of the problems facing young men. These factors need to be understood for their greater impact on adolescent males than on their female counterparts.

Boys develop both cognitively and physically at a slower rate than girls. The neurological structures contributing to reading acquisition develop at a later age for boys, leaving them at risk for falling behind their female counterparts in their academic development (Sax, 2001). Research has found that parents have a greater tendency to use physical punishment with sons rather than daughters (Garbarino, 1999). The general culture presents the message to boys that they must be tough and handle things on their own. Boys are discouraged from expressing vulnerability and from asking for help when they are struggling emotionally (Courtenay, 2001). Suicidal tendencies have historically been more difficult to diagnose in boys than in girls. Many mental health practitioners fail to diagnose a boy's serious depression because they don't realize that the young man's acting-out behaviors and substance abuse can camouflage depression as he contemplates suicide (Cochran & Rabinowitz, 2000).

Therapists must penetrate the smokescreens that conceal a young man's emotional needs and his fledgling efforts to care for himself. Too often the boys I see in therapy have had many of their needs overlooked due to their hyperactivity, substance abuse, aggression, and oppositional behavior. Frequently, the problems manifested by the young man go untreated due to cultural expectations that the boy should just "learn to handle his problems" and control the behavior altogether. The therapist easily can become frustrated trying to treat young men due to what is perceived as resistance to receiving help. The boy's refusal may be interpreted as oppositional behavior that cannot be overcome within the confines of the therapeutic relationship. The therapeutic connection may be a tenuous one due to the boy's reluctance to engage in counseling and the therapist's misinterpretation of the purpose of the boy's acting out. Some professionals unintentionally become alienated after trying to break through a boy's emotional armor, thus vitiating their ability to form a therapeutic alliance.

## STRENGTHS-BASED APPROACH TO PSYCHOTHERAPY WITH ADOLESCENT BOYS

Obviously, effectively engaging boys at the outset of psychotherapy has its own set of problems. A boy's expectations for counseling may have been diluted and influenced by cultural, familial, and social viewpoints before he even enters the therapist's office. Starting at a very young age, certain expectations of boys are dispensed by the adults in our culture. Boys are expected to constrain their emotions and never show signs of emotional weakness. The guilt and shame boys feel for their failure to contain emotions, even during times of dire adversity, will often result in a pattern of repression and withdrawal.

As noted, growing up male in today's world has a whole new set of limitations that may not have existed even 20 years ago. Being a male predisposes a boy to presuppose that he should care for his own problems without someone outside the family stepping in and making more of a "mess out of things." It is important for the therapist to help the boy reinterpret his actions and realize his true capacities and strengths. The therapist should serve as a resource for the boy to gain insight into to the process whereby he has externalized problems, such as aggression and disruption, or the process of his internalized problems, such as depression and anxiety.

Resilience is defined as the "ability to recover and adjust easily to misfortune or change" (Merriam Webster). In the field of psychology, resilience is viewed as an individual's positive adaptation when significant adversity or trauma is encountered. Resilience is considered a two-dimensional construct that incorporates a certain exposure to adversity and the accompanying positive adjustment to that adversity. Adversity is defined as risks associated with negative life conditions such as poverty, limited education, racism, bigotry, psychological trauma, and violence.

The resilience of the individual has intrigued sociologists, psychologists, and educators around the world. The question arises as to how young people have succeeded against huge odds. They have been able to overcome poverty, drug-addicted parents, homelessness, and other difficult family situations.

Sometimes the adolescent demonstrates resilience without recognizing his own strengths and capacity for change. A young person might struggle and survive under abnormally difficult conditions, yet never fully realize how he has already overcome seemingly impossible and desperate conditions. Boys have been conditioned to believe that the circumstances that they are undergoing might be bad, but they should just "suck it up" if they feel emotionally overwhelmed. Complaining to others is interpreted as being a "mama's boy" who cannot take whatever society and brutal family circumstances dish out.

Providing the young man with a framework for understanding his own strengths and defining a means of overcoming his problems can be very challenging. In therapy, it is important for the boy to describe his perception of how he came to be sitting in the therapist's office in the first place. For the most part, very few boys come to the therapy session without ascribing to someone else their reason for being there. In other words, the boy complains that he would not have considered counseling unless he had been forcefully persuaded by his school principal, probation officer, judge, or parents (most often at the insistence of his mother). The familiar refrain is that the boy's parents are "the ones who need therapy since they argue all the time about the lamest things."

Finding a way to hear a boy's personal story is a key to opening up the young man to recognizing his own strengths and resiliency. Eron and Lund (1996) refer to providing a boy with a conversation in which he describes other's perceptions of himself and the problem. It is important that the boy begin to see that his "bad" behavior might be the source of his survival and that his oppositional actions exert a powerful influence over himself and others.

When engaging young men in therapy, it is critical for the therapist to use a strengths-based approach that highlights the boy's already existing capacities. The task for the therapist and boy is to discover these strengths. I frequently explain to the boy that therapy will provide us with time to "mine" together in order to unearth his precious abilities that are often hidden below the surface.

## USEFUL CONVERSATIONS: UNDERSTANDING A FATHER'S ABSENCE

As has been recounted in the life of Barack Obama, many young men spend an inordinate portion of their lives in search of their fathers. A father who is absent, either emotionally or physically, from a son's life can have a profound impact on his growth and sense of self. Boys are often raised in father-absent homes due to the high divorce rate, the tendency of courts to award child custody to mothers, and the all-too-common social pathology of fathers abandoning their children. As a result, boys will often feel confused about what it means to be a man and they struggle to fit in without the steady guidance of their fathers (Heesacker, Baker, & Romelus, 2005).

When awaiting a family's entrance for an initial session, I have become accustomed to the familiar flurry of verbal exchanges erupting on the street outside my second-story office between a boy and his parents. Only portions of the arguments can usually be deciphered, but even though the lyrics might vary, the song has a remarkably consistent tune. The parent tries to coax the boy into the building as his protests increase among a spattering of obscenities. As the family ascends the stairs, the argument reaches a crescendo and then is followed by silence as they enter my waiting room door.

When I open my office door, the scene is invariably the same. The adolescent boy is seated in the waiting room as far away as possible from the parent, usually the mother. The mother looks up in anticipation and hopes that maybe this psychologist, this time, will be able to provide the family with some relief from the incessant tension, arguments, headaches, and frustration. The boy is slumped over in his seat with the hood of his sweatshirt pulled up over his head, intent on not looking up. The mother begins to talk for the two of them. The young man is now trapped. It is too late for him to argue any longer with his mother, and it is certainly too late for him to run out of the waiting room. I invite the two of them to come into my office.

In one particular case, a boy, Alonzo, made it abundantly clear that he was not going to talk. If there was anything to be said, it was up to his mother. He did not want to be there. Of course, what adolescent would want to see a psychologist when his friends were just down the street hanging out on the benches in front of the municipal parking lots? He had gone to school all day and was not remotely interested in listening to another adult lecture about what he should be doing with his life. The entire situation was an intrusion on his routine and his social life. Further, if anybody had a problem, it was his parents. They were the ones who were always losing their cool and arguing with him and with one another behind the closed doors of their bedroom.

The session was comprised mostly of the mother's complaints about Alonzo's impact on the family. Everything had been going reasonably well until the past year. Alonzo was a good athlete and had participated on a number of teams while in middle school. But, during the ninth grade, he had begun hanging out with the wrong type of kids. Many of them just wanted to skateboard, to play Xbox, and to smoke marijuana. On several occasions, Alonzo's mother suspected him of smoking but she could never be sure. Then she received a call from the assistant principal at the high school informing her that Alonzo had been caught with a small amount of marijuana while in gym class. He had neglected to bring a change of clothes for gym class and was caught exchanging "weed" with a friend while they sat in the stands as the other boys played basketball.

Alonzo's mother, Gabriella, burst into tears as she described the multitudinous and occasionally vicious arguments that had erupted in the last six months with her husband. She complained that her husband was in "denial" about their oldest son's problems. Her husband was frustrated and described her as being a "drama queen." Basically, he perceived Alonzo as being a good boy who was simply going through a "stage that all boys go through." In his opinion, his wife needed to lighten up. All the while, school referrals mounted for Alonzo's oppositional and disrespectful behavior at school. Gabriella felt overwhelmed by her responsibilities at work and home, so she called upon a friend whom she knew had taken her teenage son to me several years previously. Despite the overt protests of her son and the subtle protests of her husband, Alonzo's mother set up an appointment with me.

Alonzo's relationship with his father had been fractured for years. His father, Randolph, worked for a large computer company that required most of his time be spent either in the office or traveling. As his only son grew, Randolph believed that he had to make a choice between his job and his family. He simply could not keep up with both. As had been the case with his own father, Randolph relinquished his relationship with his son in favor of the daily and nightly rigors of his job. Somebody had to keep the family above water financially and surely his wife's modest salary as a schoolteacher would not keep them afloat.

I asked Alonzo if I could speak to him directly. He shrugged his shoulders and uttered a sarcastic "whatever." I offered that it was not fair to keep him out of a conversation that so clearly involved him and required his input, but first I wished to explain my personal bias regarding counseling. I realized that he did not want to be here. I wondered aloud when he ever had a chance to talk things over in a rational way with an adult. In particular, which adults (for example, a teacher, an uncle, or a mentor) did Alonzo speak with on a regular basis? It is my biased opinion that all 14- to 18-year-old boys are "knuckleheads," and candidly, I admitted I had been one myself. We "knuckleheads" just cannot get a clear picture of what our role in our family should be. We are stuck between the expectations of our parents and school and between what we really want for ourselves. Sometimes, when the pressure becomes too severe, we act foolishly. We don't know how to deal with stress. Nobody has shown us how to cope with pressure. So, we say something stupid or act badly toward our parents, girlfriends, teachers, siblings, or our friends in general. We get stuck and can't really ask anybody how to get out of our predicament, because, as a "boy-almost-man," it is assumed that we should know better. We don't know any better, of course, and we stubbornly use our little boy's ways of coping with the mature responsibilities surrounding us. Despite having just met him, I realized that Alonzo possessed a great deal of power and he could influence his family in many ways, sometimes in ways he didn't even realize. Throughout this discourse, I sought to normalize this transition point for Alonzo and to begin the process of highlighting his strengths.

As Alonzo began to look up for the first time, I further questioned, without expecting an answer, whether his father would be comfortable with me talking to his son. Most fathers don't want somebody else doing the speaking for them. I suggested that I call Randolph and invite him to my office so we could get to the bottom of this whole thing and get this counseling business over with as quickly as possible. I ventured that I preferred to avoid long drawn-out counseling meetings that might last over a course of months or, even worse, years.

It has been my experience that the absent father will subtly (or not so subtly) discourage his son from talking to another man about the family's problems. Without the father's approval, the son might continue to present his resistant front of disrespect and opposition to the counseling. It is critical for a father to provide his son with an opportunity to recognize his part in solving the family dilemma.

Now that we had heard his mother's side of the story, I suggested to Alonzo that he should encourage his father to accept my invitation and attend the next session to offer his perception about the family situation. Despite his father's likely reluctance, Alonzo should "continue to take charge" of the situation and help his father create time to meet and get things out on the table.

## CROSSING THE BRIDGE INTO MANHOOD

When Alonzo's father entered the office with his son at the second session, I complimented Alonzo for facilitating the meeting with the three of us. I informed Randolph that his son had been orchestrating this meeting for the past several months, in view of the host of acting out behaviors that he had been exhibiting both at home and school. I reiterated that I perceived Alonzo to be a "take charge" individual who must have been modeling the behavior of one or both of his parents. I noted that Alonzo is clearly at a pivotal point in his development and that his behavior was not necessarily "bad," but rather misguided. He simply was looking for guidance at this juncture in his life. This "take charge" and assertive characteristic had the potential to lead both Alonzo and his parents out of their current predicament.

Before either Randolph or Alonzo had much time to comment on my observations, I asked each for their patience in listening to my following proposal. First of all, it is important to realize that Alonzo was facing a normal developmental crossroad in his life. In today's world, there never seems to be any time to honor the respective roles that each of us possess in our families. In primitive cultures, there are rituals that are initiated to cope with what our current American culture has diagnosed as "oppositional" or "pathological" behavior. Alonzo's behavior warranted neither a psychiatric diagnosis nor the simple dismissal that his behavior reflected that "boys will be boys." His acting out was much more complex and deeply ingrained than it might appear on the surface. Perhaps we had overlooked some of the rituals that should guide his behavior. Alonzo was at a transition point and his needs might have been dismissed as he strived to become a man.

Primitive cultures frequently possess deep human wisdom and enact rituals to assist their members in moving from one stage of life to another, including birth, marriage, and death. Distinct rites of passage guide tribal members from childhood to adulthood. Margaret Mead addressed this issue in *Coming of Age in Samoa* (1973) when she expressed the idea that all children, regardless of their ethnic milieu, come to a moment during their teenage years when they begin to look beyond themselves and they become aware of the rest of society. This is a time of awakening when the adolescent begins to celebrate his gifts and looks for ways to fit into the community. At this point in development, the boy is a child no longer, nor is he yet a man. In some cultures, certain rites are established just for males to lead them to become the accomplished elders of the tribe who will someday impart their wisdom to another generation.

Each rite of passage follows a prescribed series of events. Inevitably there is an informational period punctuated with rituals that require a boy to accomplish something noteworthy to mark his transition. In the case of girls and women, there is a physiological transition point that boys and men do not experience. A girl's first menstruation marks her entry into womanhood and menopause marks her passage into a more mature stage of life. Women learn naturally about the seasons of life but men experience no clear demarcation between childhood and adulthood. To compensate, distinct rituals are created in primitive cultures for boys to experience the changes in life.

In some tribes, the father and elders of the community set aside a time to lead the boy into manhood. For the most part, the rearing of children is relegated to the women in the community. Then, in early adolescence, a boy indicates he is ready to move to the next stage in his life. Elders in the community note his intention and make preparations for the boys of the tribe to become initiated into adulthood. On one specific night in the spring, male elders go from one home to the next to select boys for initiation. The mother anticipates this ritual for her son and argues and fights with the elders. The mother dramatically contends that her adolescent boy is not ready to become a man. Often the elders pull the reluctant and sobbing boy from his home against the mother's wishes. This marks the beginning of his role as a man in the village.

There is much commotion and screaming as the mothers follow their sons and elders down the pathways of the village. Eventually, they reach the shore and a bridge leading to an island where more of the elders await the boys for the rites of passage. The mothers make one last effort to convince the elders that their sons are not ready for the passage across the bridge, but their efforts ultimately fail, and they all return to the village. In actuality, the mothers and elders had been play-acting for this rite. The mothers then return to one of the female elders' homes to drink tea and compliment each other on their Academy Award–winning performances. "I put up quite a fuss. I am sure that my son really believed that I wanted him to stay and remain a little boy."

Only the father can help the boy get across the bridge. In our culture, the forbidden acts of consuming alcohol/drugs, engaging in sex, and driving a car are seen as gateways into manhood, so few boys in our society have the opportunity for their fathers to guide them to manhood. In our modern and "sophisticated" culture, this most important life passage is treated more as an extended period of "illness." Boys will protest that they need their independence while they continue to behave in ways that guarantee their protracted dependence. This adolescent period is endured with much complaining on both sides until it mercifully passes with time. By contrast, once a tribal boy crosses the bridge, his elders engage him in a series of rituals, and he subsequently assumes the responsibilities accompanying manhood. When he returns to the village after the weekend sojourn, the boy is no longer considered by the members of his village to be a child. It is now time for him to be a responsible and contributing adult to the village.

During the course of therapy, it becomes the father's job to help his son reach manhood, no matter how much he might kick and scream while being led across to the "island." I suggested that Randolph "take charge" of a specific activity that would begin his son's initiation into manhood. At this point, I wanted to empower Randolph with taking a more active role in guiding his son through this difficult life transition. Randolph suggested that they spend a weekend "away from everything" while camping in the mountains. They had not been away together since Alonzo's days as a Cub Scout. Alonzo started to protest that his father would not follow through and that a business meeting would interfere with their plans. I suggested that Alonzo was cleverly challenging his father to "take charge" of the situation by denying his own ability to begin the process of initiation. However, Alonzo should know that his father doesn't need the impetus to initiate the rituals since this is actually a natural process that his father will undertake.

After the first camping weekend, Randolph and Alonzo admitted that they had a good time, but no magical transformation had taken place. Alonzo continued to argue with his mother and he received another referral at school for talking back to a teacher in the cafeteria. I encouraged Randolph, an elder in his family's "tribe," to counsel his son in the subsequent meetings about his responsibilities to school and family. It was important that Alonzo recognize that all future advice delivered by his father would take into consideration that he is now a young adult who is receptive to change. It was Alonzo's responsibility to "take charge" of setting up the weekly luncheon meetings at a restaurant in town so that they could share some of this time for "counsel." As a young adult, it was imperative that Alonzo set the time and place for the Saturday meetings to discuss his concerns with his father/elder. Within two months, Randolph and Alonzo decided that they no longer needed to attend therapy sessions with me as their Saturday meetings served the same purpose. Tensions in Alonzo,

Randolph, and Gabriella's home declined considerably. Throughout this period of ritual, the entire family demonstrated a creative means of promoting their own resilience and their ability to transcend old unconstructive patterns of interaction.

## THE AUDACITY TO BELIEVE

As President Obama assumes the reins of leadership in America, he serves as a constant reminder to all young men of what can be achieved when they believe in the power of their own strengths. The story of Alonzo and his family mirrors the capacity for resilience and personal power expressed in the Obama story. Alonzo struggled to avoid the pitfalls of pathology scattered along the road to his manhood. He found hope to alter his life during this period of stress and confusion. As therapists, it becomes our role to provide a palette with which a boy may begin to paint a self-portrait that accentuates his power and strengths. With these strengths discovered, no longer will the boy be lured back into a customary cycle of self-destructive pathology.

No strategic, solution-focused, or paradoxical interventions will ever be effective unless the therapist truly believes in the boy's ability to cope with his personal roadblocks. Only then can the adolescent male be armed with means for transforming pathology into strength. Once this transformation takes place, the young male can assume with audacity the hope and change he will need for entering into a healthy adulthood.

## REFERENCES

Baker, R., & King, S. E. (2004). Child sexual abuse and incest. In R. T. Francoeur & R. J. Noonan (Eds.), *International encyclopedia of sexuality* (pp. 1233–1237). New York: Continuum.

Borowsky, I. W., Ireland, M., & Resnick, M. D. (2001). Adolescent suicide attempts: Risks and protectors. *Pediatrics, 107,* 485–493.

Cochran, S. V., & Rabinowitz, F. E. (2000). *Men and depression: Clinical and empirical perspectives.* San Diego, CA: Academic Press.

Courtenay, W. H. (2001). Counseling men in medical settings: The Six-Point Health Plan. In G. R. Brooks & G. E. Good (Eds.), *The new handbook of psychotherapy and counseling with men: A comprehensive guide to setting, problems, and treatment approaches* (pp. 59–91). San Francisco: Jossey-Bass.

Eron, J., & Lund, T. (1996). *Narrative solutions in brief therapy.* New York: The Guilford Press.

Garbarino, J. (1999). *Lost Boys: Why our sons turn violent and how we can save them.* New York: Free Press.

Heesacker, M., Baker, J. O., & Romelus, E. M. (2005, August). Development of an empirically derived measure of father hunger. In J. M. Robertson (Chair), The Frontline PBS documentary *Country Boys: Theoretical and practical implications for psychologists*. Symposium conducted at the annual convention of the American Psychological Association. Washington, DC.

Mead, M. (1973). *Coming of age in Samoa: A psychological study of primitive youth for western civilization*. New York: American Museum of Natural History.

Sax, L. (2001). Reclaiming kindergarten: Making kindergarten less harmful for boys. *Psychology of Men and Masculinity, 2*, 3–12.

# 8

# Revering the Suffering and Strengths of Adolescent Girls

*Megan Barbera, Nancy Tsoubris, and Donna Zulch*

> Relationships are all there is. Everything in the universe only exists because it is in relationship to everything else. Nothing exists in isolation.
>
> —Margaret Wheatley

Ann was nine when her father shot himself in the head; Ann was the first to discover the body. In addition, Ann's mother was incarcerated on two occasions for writing bad checks and other mysterious problems before and after Ann's father's suicide. Ann lived with her aunt and uncle while her mother was incarcerated but eventually went back to live with her mother briefly. After some time she returned to her aunt and uncle and was subsequently adopted. Ann was previously seen in an outpatient child guidance clinic, and reports having had numerous therapists over the years.

As therapists, we are all too well aware that Ann's painful story is not unique. Ann and girls like her face more challenges, trauma, grief, heartache, and disconnection than most people will in a lifetime. Still other girls, without a past as traumatic as Ann's, find their way to therapy with a vast array of presenting problems, including depression, self-mutilation, anxiety, panic, substance use, delinquency, body-image issues, peer challenges, and parental conflict. These issues manifest themselves at a time when girls are entering the challenging and sometimes daunting stage of puberty. In addition, the societal challenges with which 21st-century girls are faced, such as poverty, abuse, and neglect, are compounded with the increasing sexualization of young girls. The American Psychological Association's Task Force on the Sexualization of Girls (2007) reported that this trend has a deleterious impact on a young girl's development including body shame and devaluation of their cognitive abilities. Sexualization has been shown to produce depression, low self-esteem, and eating disorders. The media, including television, movies, internet, music lyrics, video games, and advertising, all play a role in the sexualization of young girls in America.

> At puberty, a girl begins to search in earnest for outside validation for her innermost hopes and dreams for herself as a young woman. When she doesn't find what she's looking for, or when she sees women making compromises that the males in her family or society are not asked to make, she quite naturally becomes angry, frightened, or disappointed. (Northrup, 2005, p. 463)

The adolescent search for outside validation, that is validation from others besides a parent, and more specifically, her mother, is a healthy part of normal development and the beginning of the individuation process. The success of the individuation process depends greatly on the quality of the mother and child bond. Christiane Northrup (2005) speaks of the biological need a daughter has for her mother, which exists throughout her development. "Not only was our mother's body the source of life for us but it was her face that we looked to, to see how we were doing. By gazing into our mother's eyes and experiencing her response to us, we learned crucial first lessons about our own worth" (Northrup, p. 6). If this attachment is successful, adolescence can be an exciting, yet still challenging experience when the adolescent feels empowered by the love and commitment her mother has given her. But what happens when this crucial attachment does not exist or if it is severely damaged due to separation, trauma, parental limitations, or mental health issues? Oftentimes, the girls we treat have either lost this essential bond or have never experienced it, thus entering the transformative period of adolescence with a sense of disconnection, which is the breeding ground for the problems we are trying to solve.

Yet despite this disconnection, children have the extraordinary capacity to be resilient and, in fact, hardy. Resilience is the positive capacity of people to cope with stress and catastrophe. Within health psychology, the concept of hardiness (DeBold, Brown, Weseen, & Brookins, 1999) describes how people make sense of and respond to stresses in their lives. Hardiness consists of three key zones: hardiness control, hardiness challenge, and hardiness commitment. "Hardiness control" refers to the capability of making choices and using positive coping skills accordingly. "Hardiness challenge" is the ability to change at a time when one feels challenged and mobilized rather than defeated. "Hardiness commitment" describes an individual's belief system, sense of purpose, connection to others, and recognition that there are resources for one's support (DeBold et al., 1999). Yet how does a therapist faced with a child, like Ann, who has been traumatized by the abandonment of her mother and father and hiding her feces in plastic bags under her bed, discover and empower a girl's hardiness to begin the healing process?

If a therapist is to assist the adolescent in establishing a "hardiness commitment" zone, the necessary focus of therapy is to make an empowering connection to the client so that the healing work can begin. In *The Healing Connection*, Jean Baker Miller and Irene Stiver (1997) point out that the primary goal of therapy must focus on understanding sources of disconnection and move from there to a connection that is mutually empowering. From this mutual connection the client experiences a new relational experience which is vital to the healing process (Miller and Stiver, p. 121). From this new experience, the adolescent girl experiences support, encouragement, and compassion; she can competently connect to her own worth, to others and to a system of beliefs that will guide her as she resists life's stressors (DeBold et al., 1999).

## FINDING COMMON GROUND (THE PATH OF LEAST RESISTANCE)

Entering into and becoming authentically engaged in a therapeutic relationship with young girls involves a therapist's willingness to model honesty, flexibility, and unconditional positive regard. Most of our young clients pay close attention to our every nuance from the onset of therapy, observing every subtle detail and action, both verbal and nonverbal, which lays the foundation of the therapeutic relationship. As the therapist assesses clinical risk, needs, and best course of treatment, the ever-watchful adolescent girl is simultaneously gauging and testing our authenticity, fortitude, and capacity to genuinely care and serve as a trusted guide. Martha Straus (1999) points out: "In fact, the lack of strong research evidence supporting one therapeutic technique over another may be attributable to the fact that *who* we are in therapy is more important than *what* we do" (p. 38). Likewise, adolescent girls look to their therapist as a model of good self-care, appropriate emotional regulation, and purposeful self-control. Thus, it is during this early juncture in therapy when the therapist must be acutely aware of her actions as well as any potential issues that may interfere with this critical relationship-building phase. And, it is during this phase that the therapist must objectively assess the presence of a good clinical fit. In other words, if the therapist believes that, for any reason, the therapist-client match is not conducive to beneficial work, she acknowledges this in a timely and tactful manner, and then, so not to disempower, the adolescent is consulted about why another referral may be more appropriate. The teen's feedback about the "goodness of fit" between her and the therapist should be solicited and valued equally. Adolescents seek and frequently demand honesty and will only find therapeutic benefit from engaging with us in a relationship that is authentic and free of any barriers that prevent full trust and engagement.

## IDENTIFYING AND HONORING STRENGTHS

In her book *Adolescent Girls in Crisis,* Martha Straus (2007) discusses the importance of incorporating a focus on client strengths starting at the onset of therapy. "From the point of the referral onward, you'll need to be hunting down, learning all about, and helping to develop sources of competence and pleasure in girls' lives" (Straus, p. 132). While adolescents are referred from a variety of sources (rarely self-initiated) for assistance on working through one or more "presenting problems," a trusting relationship between therapist and client can become a safe haven for girls to refine, or in some cases begin, the delicate process of self-nurturing by articulating and learning to attend to their inherent abilities and strengths. For many girls, strengths-based talk therapy alone can work to elicit and solidify these feelings of validation. However, for those adolescents who do not respond to talk therapy, the attentive clinician will need to shift her treatment paradigm to incorporate other methods of forging a meaningful therapeutic connection. In such situations, it is the adolescent who serves as the guide: What are her interests? How does she prefer to spend her time? Is she better able to access her feelings nonverbally through other expressive mediums? Does she become increasingly comfortable with the therapeutic process in the absence of eye contact? How about if the clinician moves about the room providing subtle distraction? Engages in a seemingly unrelated neutral activity? Whichever approach the therapist chooses to take must attend to the unique strengths of her client, as these strengths, no matter how obscure or seemingly insignificant, serve as the first pull in the direction of tapping into one's personal power.

## WAYS OF PROMOTING RESILIENCY

In their discussion of women's self-development during adolescence, Judith Jordan, Alexandra Kaplan, Jean Baker Miller, Irene Stiver, and Janet Surrey (1991) stated the following:

> Late adolescence is an important period in the development of women's core relational self-structure. Charting the course of development during this phase involves identifying and describing the paths by which the young woman's relational self grows in complexity, flexibility, sensitivity, and adaptability. The many planes along which this growth occurs include (1) an increased potential for entering into mutually empathic relationships characterized by being able to share one's own affective states and to respond to the affect of others; (2) relational flexibility, or the capacity to permit relationships to change and evolve; (3) an ability and willingness to work through relational conflict while

> continuing to value the core of emotional connection; and (4) the capacity to feel more empowered as a result of one's inner sense of relational connection to others, particularly to mothers. (p. 131)

Hence, the therapeutic relationship can be viewed as a microcosm for the other significant relationships in a young woman's life. To this end, an emotionally safe and stable connection in therapy makes room for the adolescent to acquire and test out new relationship skills in her wider familial and social circle, a connection that can be centered on the initiation of her own needs and desires, rather than solely a self-sacrificing response to the needs of others. During this phase of therapy, the clinician provides key guidance in a number of areas. First, by providing appropriate developmental advice and being willing to utilize purposeful self-disclosure, the clinician models a relational cornerstone: reciprocal trust. Second, as the struggles of adolescent girls are often rooted in loneliness, it is important that the therapist works to normalize her experience, both to frame the resolution of any given presenting problem in a manageable light and to support her need for connection with family members and peers. In doing so, the therapist should involve as many members of the client's support system as the client willingly allows. Straus (2007) points out: "The problem here is that adolescents have too much privacy. They are yearning for more contact with their parents and with more people, but we unwittingly undermine this desire by reinforcing the distance between them and adults" (p. 129). As all relationships ultimately are, therapy is a time-limited and evolving process from which mutual learning takes place. Thus, whether we have only a few sessions or see an extended period of work to completion with a client, the lessons we help our young clients learn can and will, in some form, be generalized beyond the confines of the therapist's office. In other words, the more purposeful work we do promoting our client's strengths and honoring her search for self during this short period of time, the better the likelihood that she will be able to then find deeper and more self-nurturing connections in her relationships with others after she moves on from therapy.

What does bearing witness to the suffering of adolescent girls require of us? How do we provide her the space and safe haven for her healing to occur? We make no judgments, approaching them with reverence and support to feel and honor their pain. We help them to name and express their feelings in safe and healthy ways. Sue, a 14-year-old only child, presented in therapy following a referral from her guidance counselor to address failing grades, withdrawing behavior, and the recent breakup with her boyfriend. During the initial visit, Sue indicated that she was "unlovable" and repeatedly made references to her mother's well-being following her father's recent departure from the home. During the next several sessions, it became clear that Sue was struggling significantly with making sense of the traumatic occurrences in the family yet only expressing self-loathing and self-defeating statements. This prompted the therapist to ask Sue to bring in pictures of a family vacation. The therapist used this link to her past to elicit previously unexpressed emotions about her father's infidelity and subsequent abandonment.

*T*: Look in this mirror. What do you see?

*S*: I see pimples.

*T*: Look deeper. What might be below the skin?

*S*: I look disgusting.

*T*: Why do you think you look disgusting?

*S*: Well my boyfriend obviously thought I was.

*T*: What usually happens when people are disgusting?

*S*: People leave.

*T*: Like who?

*S*: Like Dad. He left us! He was so stupid. We were such a good family. (Sue's voice is raised and she begins to cry.) We used to go to the Jersey shore every summer. He was so stupid to do that!

*T*: Can you tell me what this feels like to you?

*S*: It makes me so angry!

*T*: Yes, you are angry! What does this anger feel like to you?

At this point, Sue stands with fists clenched and begins to sob. It is the first time Sue has connected to and verbalized her anger about her father's abandonment, facilitated by the use of the photos. By validating her feelings and leaving Sue the space to first allow the feelings to surface and share them with another, the therapist assisted her finding a new pathway for telling her story and coping with the pain of past.

In *Women's Growth and Connection* (1991), Jordan and her colleagues explained that one of the most destructive psychological phenomena is to suffer an experience and then not have the permission to experience it—that is "to know it, name it and react with the emotions that it evokes" (p. 192).

Such an experience is inevitably a social encounter; it occurs in interaction with other people. The trouble comes when powerful people surrounding you say that you cannot react that way and, more importantly, that you do not have the emotions and the perceptions that you, in fact, have. Not only do you suffer deprivation or attack per se, but you suffer the experience of complex emotions and the simultaneous "disconfirmation" of them—often followed by punishment for any attempt to express the feelings directly. Such experiences make it almost impossible to know what you are experiencing. This is terrible and confusing for adults. It is even more so for children (Jordan et al., pp. 192–193).

For Sue, being allowed to express her anger and sadness openly is an experience that many adolescent girls are not permitted. The social and cultural message often learned is that such expression is inappropriate or intolerable. Each of us can recall a time where we may have heard, "don't cry," "don't be angry," or "you shouldn't feel that way" as a child. The implied or sometimes stated message is that anger and sadness is intolerable for the adult to honor and thus intolerable for the child to experience as well. Instead of learning how to cope with this normal and natural response, the confused child not only feels invalidated but also learns to dishonor and suppress these emotions as insignificant, unhealthy, and unacceptable. In the example of Sue, the therapist provided Sue with a strategy which strengthened Sue's ability to explore the complex emotions and then the permission to express them. By bearing witness with reverence to Sue's outpouring of emotions, the therapist facilitated a healing experience for Sue that she could build upon and then generalize to relationships outside the realm of the therapeutic setting.

Creating rituals or ceremonies is another way that a therapist can incorporate reverence into the healing process. In *Rituals in Family and Family Therapy*, Imber-Black, Roberts, and Whiting (2003) described the use of a ritual as an opportunity to promote a change in the life of an individual or family or social group. In the therapeutic framework, a ritual can be used to "bring about a change, such as the solving of a problem or the healing of a wound" (p. 160). The essential elements in creating a ritual with children are that it reflects the child's worldview and that it is developmentally appropriate. These elements make the ritual believable to the child and thus can affect change. In the following case study, the therapist used the ritual to facilitate the expression of deep sadness that Ann, the adolescent we described at the beginning of the chapter, felt. Ann, at the age of 14, is speaking about a letter she wrote to her deceased grandfather.

*T*: How did you do with the letter, Ann?

*A*: I wrote it. I can't believe I wrote it!

*T*: Wow! Sounds like you surprised yourself.

*A*: I did. (Ann starts to cry.)

*T*: If your tears could talk, what would they say?

*A*: My grandpa is dead. I can't ever see him again. He left money for me and Gary though, for doctors and stuff. He really loved us a lot.

*T*: Sounds like you really miss him so much and that he was good to you and Gary and wanted to make sure you were taken care of. Did you ever get to say good-bye to him?

*A*: No. No. Nobody even seemed to think it mattered to us!

*T*: Is there any way you could say goodbye to him now, do you think?

*A*: I don't know. (She holds her face and looks like she is thinking very hard.)

*A*: I don't know. I can't think of anything. But I would want him to hear me from Heaven.

*T*: Well, Heaven is pretty far up in the air. I wonder how you could let him know. Hmmm.

*A*: (She smiles.) I know!

*T*: What?

*A*: Maybe we could send up a balloon? Like a message in a bottle thing.

*T*: That is some idea! I could get a helium balloon for our next visit. Would that work?

*A*: Yes! Could you get a blue one please, that's his favorite color.

*T*: OK. That will be my assignment. What will you do?

*A*: I will put down everything I want to tell him on a piece of paper. Can we send that up with it?

*T*: Sounds like a plan to me. I will bring some string. Where should we launch it from?

*A*: Can we go out there? (She points out the window to the back yard behind the office.)

We ceremoniously sent the balloon up to Heaven the next week. She told the therapist at the start of the session she wanted to read what she wrote before we launched it. This is what she shared:

I am really sorry, Pop-Pop, for all the times Gary and I called you Oscar the Grouch and made fun of you. You and Uncle Sal were like boulders for Gary and I through all the mess. You were always there. You loved us both unconditionally and for a while we treated you like crap! I am really sorry because all you wanted was to make us happy and now that you're no longer here I can't tell you that myself. You were one person who had never come into my life just to drift away. You were always there for me in your own way and I hope you know how much I miss you and Mum Mum, because you are both wonderful people and you deserved more love than I can ever give you. So, I miss you and I love you and I am sorry and good-bye. Ann.

Ann had never talked about this before. Her written letter, prepared for the balloon launching, pulled on a strength that was clear from the start: her ability, when she felt safe, to use language to clearly express her innermost feelings. She had made her amends. She said her good-byes. We revisited this once again about a month later. Ann labeled it the "apology ceremony" when we talked about the day she let the balloon go up into the air. That day she decided to do more writing and was able to use the balloon ritual repeatedly throughout her work to come to terms with her losses.

## ENDING THE THERAPEUTIC RELATIONSHIP

Just as our work with each client is unique in its content and progress, so is the ending of the therapeutic relationship. While the ideal ending with adolescents is one which is timely, planned, and discussed from the onset, attrition rates (in child therapy) range from approximately 30 to 70 percent (Kazdin, 1996; Novick, Benson, & Rembar, 1981). Thus, we must remain flexible and creative in our attempt to bring meaningful closure to the therapist-client relationship, despite any number of factors which can influence the terms under which termination occurs. Martha Straus (1999) delineates three primary causal factors of premature termination: child and family reasons (ranging from moving to unrealistic parental expectations), therapist reasons, and environmental reasons such as managed care limitations and/or case collaboration barriers. To minimize the occurrence of premature termination, Straus emphasizes the importance of the therapist being sensitive to the needs of the family system by creating a strong alliance and avoiding excessive therapy.

When planned, termination provides the final and arguably most important phase of the therapeutic relationship. It is during this phase that we can engage our clients in a healthy and heartfelt good-bye, free of the unresolved feelings surrounding loss that often accompany them into therapy. By creating an individualized, client-centered plan for termination, we, with the help of our clients, bring about a predictable, mutually agreed upon, and meaningful ending. Whether our clients leave us with the preferred "open-door option of returning to therapy" or with the knowledge that the visit will be the final one, we can support them as they move through this rite of passage by offering a simple ritual or gesture to honor their work and courage to let us in. David Epston and Michael White (1992) describe how rites of passage enable clients to:

> negotiate the passage from novice to veteran, from client to consultant. Rather than instituting a dependency on the "expert knowledge" presented by the therapist and other authorities, this therapy enables persons to arrive at a point where they can take recourse to liberating alternatives and "special" knowledge that they have resurrected and/or generated during therapy. (p. 280)

In the therapeutic collaboration with adolescent girls, we hopefully offer the reverence of the therapeutic relationship at it best. Adolescent girls in our culture from a young age repeatedly receive devaluing messages that essentially tell them that they are valued primarily for looking sexy and appealing to boys (American Psychological Association, 2007). These young women were not treated with reverence in our culture. If these devaluing and demeaning messages have not been countered by parents and other influential adults in their lives they arrive at our office door wounded by this narrow and unjust definition of self that many will have internalized. Reverence in the therapeutic relationship is the beginning of offering them an opportunity to value the unique person each one is, and to greatly expand the definition of self to include the qualities that each can rightly cherish that have nothing to do with looks or sex appeal, such as intelligence; warmth; empathy; a nice smile; academic, musical, and creative talents; and abilities in sports, to name just a few. We honor the unique essence of each girl by opening our hearts to be present with them fully in the expression of the pain and suffering. We do this to encourage the resilience that emerges from a space where trust and caring are offered and with interventions that honor each adolescent's courage to heal by reverently acknowledging their story in its unedited entirety, and their unique and special way of sharing it.

## REFERENCES


American Psychological Association. (2007). *Report of the APA task force on the sexualization of girls*. Washington, DC: American Psychological Association.

DeBold, E., Brown, L. M., Weseen, S., & Brookins, G. K. (1999). *Cultivating hardiness zones for adolescent girls: A reconceptualization of resilience in relationships with caring adults*. In N. G. Johnson, M. Roberts, & J. Worell, *Beyond appearance: A new look at adolescent girls* (pp. 181–204). Washington, DC: American Psychological Association.

Epston, D., & White, M. (1992). *Experience, contradiction, narrative, and imagination: Selected papers of David Epston & Michael White 1989–1991*. Adelaide, Australia: Dulwich Centre Publications.

Imber-Black, E., Roberts, J., & Whiting, R. A. (2003). *Rituals in families and family therapy*. New York: Norton.

Jordan, J. V., Kaplan, A. G., Miller, J. B., Stiver, I. P., & Surrey, J. L. (1991). *Women's growth in connection*. New York: The Guilford Press.

Kazdin, A. (1996). Dropping out of child psychotherapy: Issues for research and implications for practice. *Clinical Child Psychology and Psychiatry, 1*(1), 133–156.

Miller, J. B., & Stiver, I. P. (1997). *The healing connection: How women form relationships in therapy and in life*. Boston: Beacon Press.

Northrup, C. (2005). *Mother-daughter wisdom: Creating a legacy of physical and emotional health*. New York: Bantam Dell.

Novick, J., Benson, R., & Rembar, J. (1981). Patterns of termination in an outpatient clinic for children and adolescents. *Journal of the American Academy for Child Psychiatry, 20*, 833–844.

Straus, M. B. (1999). *No-talk therapy for children and adolescents*. New York: Norton.

Straus, M. B. (2007). *Adolescent girls in crisis*. New York: Norton.

# 9

# A Strengths-Based Approach to Working with Abused and Traumatized Children

*Sueann G. Kenney-Noziska*

> What lies behind us and what lies before us are small matters compared to what lies within us.
>
> —Ralph Waldo Emerson

When I first began my career, I was told that if I was on the wrong track in therapy, the child would let me know. The notion of a child "correcting" me in my therapeutic work seemed strange. However, children do indeed speak up. Countless times during play therapy sessions, children have "corrected" me by saying such things as, "That's not what's happening" or "He's not saying that." Even children with some of the most horrific and unbearable histories are able to "correct" me when I'm on the wrong therapeutic track. How is that possible? How can a traumatized child who can barely make it through the day without resorting to extreme acting-out behaviors have the strength to know when their therapist is out-of-touch with what they need?

In part, this is the beauty of utilizing a strengths-based approach when working with traumatized children—acknowledging and honoring the fact that these children are survivors with strength and determination beyond what most can imagine. They bring these strengths and skills with them into therapy and utilizing these attributes can be a vital component to the therapeutic process.

Alas, there is danger in this as well. In recognizing strengths, we must tread in a manner which does not invalidate the suffering and anguish these young ones have experienced. The challenge is to recognize, honor, and utilize the child's strengths without trivializing the suffering they have endured.

## STRENGTHS-BASED APPROACH TO PSYCHOTHERAPY WITH ABUSED AND TRAUMATIZED CHILDREN

Berg and Steiner (2003) assert that many members of the clinical population may benefit from a strengths-based approach, including those who are trauma survivors. The challenge is not to only see strengths or to distort the child's history and experiences into a positive perspective but to be sensitive to the pain while, at the same time, recognizing the skills and resources the child possesses. The strengths/competency-based approach has received increased emphasis in family therapy as well as the mental health field in general over the last decade (Allison et al., 2003). It is increasingly used in the juvenile justice system in treating both male and female adolescent offenders (Clark, 1998; Corcoran, 1997; Johnson, 2003; Pepi, 1997; Querimit & Conner, 2003), in residential treatment and inpatient treatment of children and adolescents (Nickerson, Salamone, Brooks, & Colby, 2004; LeBel et al., 2004), and in the treatment of children and youth presenting with a wide range of clinical problems (Corcoran, 2005; Helton & Smith, 2004).

A strengths-based approach with abused and traumatized children can be used as an adjunct to support more traditional approaches to therapy versus replacing these approaches. As a part of this process, the strengths of the child are assessed and used to foster healing. It is an approach that seeks to actively and deliberately use strengths, resources, and previous successes to create a foundation for therapy and to develop future growth despite the circumstances or events of the child's past. The therapist is invested in both building on strengths as well as repairing abuse and trauma.

## CASE EXAMPLE: SAMANTHA

Samantha is an eight-year-old African American female who has experienced multiple traumatic and abusive events. Samantha's mother was a chronic substance abuser who was neglectful as well as emotionally and physically abusive. When Samantha was five years of age, her mother abandoned her in a known drug house where she was subjected to sexual abuse and other horrors. It is believed Samantha lived under these conditions for six to eight months until the house was raided by authorities and Samantha was taken into protective custody. Neither Samantha's mother nor father could be located and, in absence of a viable relative placement, she bounced from foster home to foster home. Samantha oscillated between being verbally and physically aggressive to peers and adults and being clingy, needy, and regressed.

Samantha entered treatment with a tough exterior but displayed an amazing capacity to engage in creative play. Although guarded, she also appeared open to the concept of trusting the therapist despite the fact she had experienced disappointment and betrayal at the hands of most adults who had entered her life. These strengths were duly noted by the therapist. In what could have been viewed as "resistance," from a strengths-based perspective, Samantha's hesitancy was viewed as a needed measure to shield her from harm. Samantha had all the reason in the world not to trust another adult in the revolving door of her life.

A strengths-based approach was employed as an adjunct to integrated play therapy constructs including Object Relations Play Therapy (Benedict, 2006), Cognitive-Behavioral Play Therapy (Knell, 2009), and Trauma-Focused Play Therapy (Gil, 2006). Directive play-based techniques were incorporated throughout treatment to help identify and utilize strengths as well as facilitate the development of a positive self-esteem. The integration of these approaches allowed a metamorphosis to occur for Samantha.

Trust and rapport were difficult to establish. However, a breakthrough occurred using a play-based intervention entitled "All Tied Up" in which Samantha was viewed as a "survivor" and reactions to abusive and traumatic events were normalized (Kenney-Noziska, 2008b). This was intriguing to Samantha and, possibly for the first time in her life, she was introduced to the concept that she possessed strengths and other positive attributes. This created a foundation from which we began exploring things Samantha had survived and the strengths she possessed. "A Mountain of Strengths" (Crenshaw, 2006) was employed as an evocative strategy whereby Samantha was invited to identify talents, strengths, and personal attributes as a part of each session. Through the intervention "I Am So Much More," Samantha was able to share aspects of herself beyond her victimization and the loss and disappointment she had experienced. Using humor and an emphasis on resiliency, the therapist was able to connect with a part of Samantha that allowed for a softening of her tough facade. Hope and optimism arose as Samantha tapped deeper into her own strengths using interventions such as "Picking Up the Pieces" during which Samantha identified her active role in "picking up the pieces" of what felt like a shattered life.

As treatment progressed, Samantha was able to explore the deep sense of sadness she had experienced at the hands of her mother who abandoned her. In addition, she began processing and integrating her history of abuse and trauma. Play themes progressed and began to include elements of protection, healing, and resolution.

As treatment came to a close, Samantha was no longer the vulnerable, victimized child she once was. She was stronger, more confident, and hopeful. Through "My Neighborhood Helpers," she was able to identify safety within her community. Safety within her own support system was additionally identified through a strengths-based intervention entitled "Lifesavers" (Kenney-Noziska, 2008b). During her final session, Samantha's progress and growth in treatment were reviewed and acknowledged using the intervention "From Start to Finish," an activity in which Samantha described her path from victim to survivor by identifying personal strengths and resources.

Samantha left treatment with a positive view of others and optimism which I have rarely experienced. No longer was she a victim—she was a strong survivor with hopes and aspirations for her future. Not only did she know her strengths and recognize her own resilience, she embraced and exuded these qualities in a way that will surely serve her in the future.

Samantha's case exemplifies how incorporating a strengths-based approach within other theoretical frameworks can be successfully utilized throughout the treatment process. The integration of these methods within the therapeutic relationship allowed Samantha to recognize and utilize her strengths and inner resources to achieve mastery over her abusive and traumatic experiences and create a life narrative that was coherent and meaningful.

## CASE EXAMPLE: CHARLES

Charles is a 14-year-old African American male who has been the victim of chronic childhood abuse and neglect. While living with his mother, a polysubstance abuser whose drug of choice was crack cocaine, Charles was sexually abused by his stepfather for a period of seven years. The abuse was extensive and included oral copulation and sodomy. Charles also experienced general neglect, exposure to domestic violence, and physical abuse. Charles was eventually placed in protective custody and his mother enrolled in a substance abuse treatment program. While in the foster care system, Charles had multiple placements. In one placement, Charles was victimized by a foster father who also perpetrated sexual abuse onto him.

Upon mother's completion of her substance abuse program, Charles was returned to her care. By this time, it appeared as if Charles's soul was incredibly damaged by the victimization he had endured. Almost immediately upon reunification, Charles began to display extreme emotional and behavioral problems. He was encopretic and would play in his feces. In addition, his mood was angry and irritable with physical aggression including punching holes in walls, slapping and hitting his mother, and beating up his younger siblings, as well as verbal aggression including intense and prolonged episodes of screaming, yelling, and using obscene and profane language.

With Charles's extensive history of abuse, his self-concept was injured and he was very leery of the intentions and motives of those around him. He was almost hypervigilant during sessions, noting every sound outside the room, and appeared preoccupied with whether the therapist was trying to "trick" him in some way. More traditional models of counseling might have been insufficient at making headway in forming a strong therapeutic relationship and in addressing the issues pertinent to treatment. As a result, therapeutic work with Charles used an integrated model which included a strengths-based approach incorporated into humanistic and cognitive-behavioral frameworks.

Charles entered treatment justifiably guarded and mistrusting. As opposed to viewing these characteristics as defensiveness or lack of motivation, they were identified as strategies he used to protect himself from being hurt and exploited by others. One way this was communicated was through the activity "Play Genogram" (Gil, 2006). During this play therapy intervention, Charles was directed to select figures to represent his thoughts and feelings about each person in his family. What was most interesting was his selection of a soldier and porcupine to represent himself. As each character was discussed, the therapist began to make connections between Charles's positive qualities and qualities of the miniatures. Charles discussed the porcupine's ability to protect itself by keeping others at a distance using its quills. As this was processed, the therapist highlighted how Charles was also able to keep others at a safe distance. Charles appeared to resonate with this and displayed insight as he discussed how his encopresis and aggression created safety and protection by ensuring that others did not get close enough to hurt him. From there, Charles processed how brave the solider was to fight wars and made a connection with his own bravery in fighting "wars" against sexual and physical abuse.

Building on Charles's strengths allowed the therapeutic relationship to grow. Eventually, the emotions underlying his anger and aggression were processed. Active coping strategies to reduce distress were developed as were cognitive coping strategies to develop more adaptive ways of viewing problems and issues. Despite Charles's severe early childhood neglect, he proved to be quite creative and artistic. These areas, in turn, became strategies that were employed to provide outlets to reduce and manage emotional distress at a more tolerable level; before it reached the peak of aggression.

As a part of developing cognitive coping strategies, specific maladaptive cognitions pertaining to Charles's self-concept were explored using the activity "Don't Lose Your Marbles." As distorted cognitions were identified, challenged, and replaced with more accurate, adaptive cognitions, an emphasis was placed on identifying strengths. The distorted cognition, "People want to use and hurt me," was challenged using Charles's ability to trust the therapist and several teachers. The final reframe created was, "There are safe people who can earn my trust and will treat me right."

Building on the metaphor of the porcupine's quills, Charles's need to protect himself from others was reexamined. During "The Wall" (Hobday

& Ollier, 2006), encopretic and aggressive behaviors which were once functional were viewed as being ineffective as they also created a barrier between Charles and those he could trust, cared about him, and wanted to help him.

As this work unfolded, Charles reached a place where he felt safe enough to create a narrative of his abusive and traumatic experiences. During this piece of therapeutic work, distorted cognitions of guilt, blame, and responsibility that significantly contributed to his low self-worth were challenged and addressed.

Work with Charles's mother was pivotal to his healing process. As opposed to viewing the mother as a "bad," abusive, and neglectful parent, a strengths-based approach connected with her desire to protect and help her son. Truly a woman who appeared to have benefited from her own treatment, a clear strength was his mother's willingness to accept responsibility for the abuse and neglect Charles had endured. To take advantage of this resource, the therapist and Charles included the mother in several early sessions. During these times, Charles's mother gave him permission to openly share the history of abuse and trauma he had endured while in her care. She sincerely apologized for the harm and brutality he had suffered and expressed amazement at his ability to survive amid such adversity. For a mother who possessed only a 9th grade education, she was articulate and succinct as she shared her own decision to turn to substances to numb out her pain and praised Charles for his ability to remain steadfast in not resorting to substance abuse to escape his past. With ease and grace, Charles's mother shared the strengths and resiliency she observed in her son. During one session, as his mother described him as brave, courageous, and strong, Charles's eyes filled with tears. It was as if his wall of defenses was beginning to crack and crumble before our eyes.

Incorporation of a strengths-based approach with Charles greatly enhanced the ability for therapeutic change and growth to occur. Working with the assets of both Charles and his mother, a foundation was created from which a strong therapeutic alliance was formed, resistance was reduced, and motivation for change increased. Without this foundation, exploring, processing, and integrating his history of abuse and trauma might not have occurred.

Although the family continued to struggle with other psychosocial stressors that often accompany multiproblem families living in low socioeconomic status, Charles reached a point where he was no longer encopretic or verbally and physically aggressive. His mood stabilized and he was able to engage in daily activities without his history of abuse serving as a trigger for maladaptive behaviors and defenses. Charles emerged from treatment with a different experience of himself and others.

## DISCUSSION AND CLINICAL IMPLICATIONS

Clinical work with abused and traumatized children is likely one of the most challenging journeys a therapist can embark on. This work requires the therapist to bear witness to harrowing and disturbing histories of victims of childhood trauma and abuse. Yet, in this work, the therapist also has the honor and privilege of working with incredibly courageous and resilient individuals.

Traumatic and abusive events are experienced differently by each child. Traumatic experiences are highly influenced by contextual factors and, subsequently, complex and heterogeneous clinical profiles emerge in our practices. There is no specific victim profile for the abused and traumatized children we encounter. Likewise, there is no one particular treatment which works for every single child. The consensus in the field of abuse and trauma is that abusive and traumatic experiences must be addressed (Cohen, Mannarino, & Deblinger, 2006; Gil 2006; Ross & O'Carroll, 2004). How this task is accomplished becomes a point of debate. There is significant evidence and support for the use of Trauma-Focused Cognitive Behavioral Therapy (TF-CBT) when working with abused and traumatized children (Cohen et al., 2006). An integrated approach which incorporates evidence-based, directive, and nondirective models may also be effective in addressing the diverse needs of this population (Gil, 2006; Gil & Jalazo, 2009; Shelby & Felix, 2005). From a play therapy perspective, there is growing support for combining different theoretical models in a clinically grounded, integrated manner to address the needs of children impacted by abuse and trauma (Gil, 2006; Kelly & Odenwalt, 2006; Kenney-Noziska, 2008a). The emphasis is placed on responding to the child's needs versus strict allegiance to one theoretical school of thought. Being responsive to the child and adapting the therapeutic approach according to the child's needs becomes essential and creates the context from which the therapist operates (Gil, 2006). While theoretical approaches may differ, treatment protocols reflecting current best practices typically include the following key elements.

### Safety

Establishing a safe environment in the therapy office (Kelly & Odenwalt, 2006), as well as a therapeutic environment conducive to expressing attributions of self-blame (Feiring, Miller-Johnson, & Cleland, 2007), are essential for the success of treatment with this population. Accomplishing this with children who have been disregarded or harmed at the very hands of those who are supposed to love and cherish them proves difficult as these children often enter treatment suspicious and uncertain about adults. The primary tools of establishing safety are to build a strong therapeutic alliance, strengthening coping resources, and to be sensitive to issues of timing and pacing as described next.

### Therapeutic Alliance

Establishing a strong therapeutic relationship, one of the most formative processes of therapy, can pose a challenge when working with abused and traumatized children. The therapeutic relationship is well-known as a factor related to therapeutic efficacy and effectiveness (Roberts & Yeager, 2006). However, for children who have experienced abusive and traumatic events, the importance of the therapeutic relationship is paramount and becomes a preliminary treatment consideration.

### Pacing, Timing, and Coping Resources

Therapy needs to move forward but with sensitivity to issues of safety and respect for the child's pace (Crenshaw, 2006). Crucial to sensitive pacing is ensuring the child possesses adequate coping strategies prior to processing abusive and traumatic information. Assessing and enhancing coping is paramount to ensure the child has the coping resources necessary to manage recalling traumatic and abusive material and deal with the anxiety, stress, and fear likely to arise during this work (Deblinger & Heflin, 1996; Kenney-Noziska, 2008a; Ross & O'Carroll, 2004). To begin trauma work without coping resources being assessed and strengthened could create an iatrogenic effect in which the intervention does harm.

### Caregiver Involvement

Involving parents as partners in therapy is a cornerstone of working with children. In the area of abuse and trauma, the literature is clear that working with parents is essential (Cohen, Mannarino, & Deblinger, 2006; Kenney-Noziska, 2008a; Shelby & Felix, 2005). However, engaging an abusive parent can be a challenge. As John Sharry (2004) states, from a strengths-based perspective, the therapist must avoid falling into the pitfalls of colluding with the abusive parent by avoiding or failing to confront the abuse and condemning, blaming, or judging the parent. Sharry (2004) additionally suggests that therapists strive to collaborate with the parent to protect the child and increase safety by joining respectfully with the parent while, at the same time, being open and honest regarding the abuse as well as mandated child protective reporting responsibilities.

Abusive parents can play a powerful role in their child's healing even though this may seem counterintuitive. When an abusive parent apologizes for the abuse they inflicted, takes responsibility for their behavior, acknowledges the child's bravery in disclosing the abuse, or recognizes the child's courage to address their traumatic past in therapy, it can be incredibly healing. By trying to understand what the parent has done right rather than focusing solely on the parent's abusive behavior, a strengths-based approach creates the potential to engage parents in therapy, overcome resistance, and may result in future abusive behavior decreasing (Anderson, 2000).

### Countertransference

In the area of abuse and trauma, the therapist is taxed with dealing constructively with child abuse and childhood trauma. This involves forming a therapeutic alliance with abusive parents, being present and bearing witness to the horrors the child has suffered, and being present with families as they embark on a potentially tumultuous process of healing. Managing countertransference through self-awareness, understanding personal reactions, and attempting to respond to these influences in a constructive manner must be confronted in a purposeful way. Due to the emotionally charged reactions that inevitably arise in working with the abuse of children, it is essential that therapists seek consultation with colleagues, supervision from more experienced and knowledgeable clinicians in the field, and aggressively pursue opportunities for continuing education in the field of child trauma.

### Self-Care

Another important, yet often overlooked issue is the inevitable stress inherent in work with abuse and trauma. The therapist is vicariously exposed to unimaginable trauma, horrifying recollections, and dehumanizing experiences. The therapist must be empathic, caring, and present without becoming engulfed in the child's trauma. Even the most seasoned therapist is not immune to the unavoidable toll this stress can take and, subsequently, self-care is paramount.

## UNIQUE ADVANTAGES OF THE STRENGTHS-BASED APPROACH IN TRAUMA WORK

A strong therapeutic relationship is an important component in work with abused and traumatized children (Ross & O'Carroll, 2004) and arguably provides a reparative experience (Gil, 2006; Kelly & Odenwalt, 2006). A strengths-based approach allows us to establish a therapeutic relationship with more ability to support and facilitate change as we highlight strengths, assets, and focus on what is "right." Honoring the child's strengths may allow us to form a stronger therapeutic relationship than we would if we operated from the perspective of looking for deficits only. While considering diagnosis, pathology, symptoms, and impairment, we also recognize strengths and resilience from the first moment the child enters our office. From this vantage point, even the child's willingness and ability to trust the therapist after betrayal, disappointment, and harm at the hands of a trusted adult is viewed as a strength.

Strengths-based assessment offers practitioners a way to assess skills, competencies, and adaptive characteristics of individuals and families. In addition, when therapists focus on strengths, they are more likely to involve and, subsequently, engage families and children in treatment (Epstein et al., 2003). The empowerment a strengths-based perspective creates may put the child in a better position to explore their abusive and traumatic experiences. As the child describes their problems and struggles, the therapist listens for strengths, skills, and resources. These things should be communicated to the child and caregiver (Sharry, 2004). The therapist is interested in how the child has coped with their traumatic experiences, not just in the damage the trauma has caused. From a strengths-based approach, the therapist works to help the child understand how they have managed to survive and uses this to continue supporting the child's ability to help themselves (Saleebey, 1992).

## CONCLUSION

A strengths-based perspective honors the resources and power of the child to heal within the context of the therapeutic environment. In this regard, a skilled therapist will strive for a balance between an overly focused conceptualization on deficits, symptoms, and damage and a "sugar-coated" conceptualization emphasizing only skills, resources, and strengths without regarding the child's history of abuse and trauma. This means acknowledging the good, the bad, and the ugly; not forsaking one for the other.

Although abusive and traumatic events impact children in profound ways; likewise, therapy can impact children in profound ways—ways that are positive, healing, and curative. My work with Samantha, Charles, and children like them has given me my deep belief that the work we do truly shapes the lives of children. However, we do not do this work alone. I am often moved by the strengths these children possess. In many ways, Samantha and Charles are more courageous than most people I know. My work with them and countless others has given me a true appreciation for recognizing strengths, resources, and resilience. Although not all cases are as successful as Samantha's and Charles's, when they are, what a joy it is for both child and therapist alike.

Utilizing a strengths-based approach in work with abuse and trauma has opened my eyes to the true courage and strength children possess. Some of the most important lessons in my career are not those that I've learned in class, seminars, or conferences, but are lessons learned from the littlest of survivors—how to endure and overcome adversity, how to persevere even when you feel alone, how to be trusting even after you've been hurt. Relationships with Samantha, Charles, and the resilient children like them are the most valuable and rewarding parts of my career. If I only carry the smallest portion of inner strength, courage, and resolve they possess, I will live a better life for it.

## REFERENCES

Allison, S., Stacey, K., Dadds, V., Roeger, L., Wood, A., & Martin, G. (2003). What the family brings: Gathering evidence for strengths-based work. *Journal of Family Therapy, 25*, 263–284.

Anderson, E. A. (2000). Views of females participating in strength based couples therapy for domestic violence. Unpublished thesis, Virginia Polytechnic Institute and State University, Blacksburg, Virginia.

Benedict, H. E. (2006). Object relations play therapy: Applications to attachment problems and relational trauma. In C. E. Schaefer & H. G. Kaduson (Eds.), *Contemporary play therapy: Theory, research, and practice* (pp. 3–27). New York: Guilford Press.

Berg, I. K., & Steiner, T. (2003). *Children's solution work*. New York: W. W. Norton & Company.

Clark, M. D. (1998). Strengths-based practice: The ABC's of working with adolescents who don't want to work with you. *Federal Probation, 62*, 46–53.

Cohen, J. A., Mannarino, A. P., & Deblinger, E. (2006). *Treating trauma and traumatic grief in children and adolescents*. New York: Guilford Press.

Corcoran, J. (1997). A solution-oriented approach to working with juvenile offenders. *Child and Adolescent Social Work Journal, 14*, 277–288.

Corcoran, J. (2005). *Building strengths and skills: A collaborative approach to working with clients*. New York: Oxford University Press.

Crenshaw, D. A. (2006). *Evocative strategies in child and adolescent psychotherapy*. Lanham, MD: Jason Aronson.

Deblinger, E., & Heflin, A. H. (1996). *Treating sexually abused children and their nonoffending parents: A cognitive behavioral approach*. Thousand Oaks, CA: Sage Publications.

Epstein, M., Harniss, M., Robbins, V., Wheeler, L., Cyrulik, S., Kriz, M., & Nelson, R. (2003). Strength-based approaches to assessment in schools. In M. D. Weist, S. W. Evan, & N. A. Lever (Eds.), *Handbook of school mental health: Advancing practice and research* (pp. 285–300). New York: Springer.

Feiring, C., Miller-Johnson, S., & Cleland, C. M. (2007). Potential pathways from stigmatization and internalizing symptoms to delinquency in sexually abused youth. *Child Maltreatment, 12*(3), 220–232.

Gil, E. (2006). *Helping abused and traumatized children: Integrating directive and nondirective approaches.* New York: Guilford Press.

Gil, E., & Jalazo, N. (2009). An illustration of science and practice: Strengthening the whole through its parts. In A. A. Drewes (Ed.), *Blending play therapy with cognitive behavioral therapy: Evidence-based and other effective treatments and techniques* (pp. 41–68). Hoboken, NJ: John Wiley & Sons.

Helton, L. R., & Smith, M. K. (2004). *Mental health practice with children and youth: A strengths and well-being model.* New York: The Haworth Press.

Hobday, A., & Ollier, K. (2006). *Creative therapy with children & adolescents.* Atascadero, CA: Impact Publishers.

Johnson, N. G. (2003). On treating adolescent girls: Focus on strengths and resiliency in psychotherapy. *Journal of Clinical Psychology, 59,* 1193–1203.

Kelly, M. M., & Odenwalt, H. C. (2006). Treatment of sexually abused children. In C. E. Schaefer & H. G. Kaduson (Eds.), *Contemporary play therapy: Theory, research, and practice* (pp. 186–211). New York: Guilford Press.

Kenney-Noziska, S. (2008a). The sexual abuse literature & considerations for play therapists. *Association for Play Therapy Mining Report, October 2008,* 1–3.

Kenney-Noziska, S. (2008b). *Techniques-techniques-techniques: Play-based activities for children, adolescents, and families.* West Conshohocken, PA: Infinity Publishing.

Knell, S. M. (2009). Cognitive-behavioral play therapy: Theory and applications. In A. A. Drewes (Ed.), *Blending play therapy with cognitive behavioral therapy: Evidence-based and other effective treatments and techniques* (pp. 117–133). Hoboken, NJ: John Wiley & Sons.

LeBel, J., Stomberg, N., Duckworth, K., Kerzner, J., Goldstein, M., and Weekes, G., et al. (2004). Child and adolescent inpatient restraint reduction: A state initiative to promote strength-based care. *Journal of the American Academy of Child & Adolescent Psychiatry, 43,* 37–45.

Nickerson, A. B., Salamone, F. J., Brooks, J. L., and Colby, S. A. (2004). Promising approaches to engaging families and building strengths in residential treatment. *Residential Treatment for Children & Youth, 22,* 1–18.

Pepi, C. L. (1997). Children without childhoods: A feminist intervention strategy utilizing systems theory and restorative justice in treating female adolescent offenders. *Women & Therapy, 20,* 85–101.

Querimit, D. S., & Conner, L. C. (2003). Empowerment psychotherapy with adolescent females of color. *Journal of Clinical Psychology, 59,* 1215–1224.

Roberts, A. R., & Yeager, K. R. (Eds.). (2006). *Foundations of evidence-based social work practice.* New York: Oxford University Press.

Ross, G., & O'Carroll, P. (2004). Cognitive behavioural psychotherapy intervention in childhood sexual abuse: Identifying new direction from the literature. *Child Abuse Review, 13*(1), 51–64.

Saleebey, D. (1992). *The strengths perspective in social work practice.* New York: Longman Publishing.

Sharry, J. (2004). *Counseling children, adolescents, and families*. London: Sage Publications.

Shelby, J. S., & Felix, E. D. (2005). Posttraumatic play therapy: The need for an integrated model of directive and nondirective approaches. In L. A. Reddy, T. M. Files-Hall, & C. E. Schaefer (Eds.), *Empirically based play interventions for children* (pp. 79–103). Washington, DC: American Psychological Association.

# 10

# A Competence Approach to Therapy with Families with Multiple Problems

*Edith C. Lawrence and Amanda F. Sovik-Johnston*

> I've learned that people will forget what you said, people will forget what you did, but people will never forget how you made them feel.
>
> —Maya Angelou

When deciding how best to help children and families seeking therapy, it is important to take into account that research consistently indicates that the family or primary caregiver is critical to children's successful long-term outcomes. In fact, some have suggested that "from the existing research, it could easily be argued that targeting family issues is the single most important point of intervention for children and adolescents" (Henggeler, Schoenwald, Borduin, Rowland, & Cunningham, 1998, as cited in Stormshak & Dishion, 2002, p. 201). Adopting a family focus to intervention may be especially critical for children living in families with multiple problems, although the work can present a special challenge for the therapist.

Typically, such families have several serious issues (e.g., poverty, abuse, mental illness), any one of which may create great stress. The problems are often complex, interactive, and multidetermined. For instance, while a child's poor conduct at school may be most proximately related to his attention deficits, his difficulties in the classroom are likely exacerbated when the parents are also struggling with inadequate housing, underemployment, and a history of substance use. Not only must the therapist assess each individual problem and its ramifications, but also recognize the interplay between these often seemingly disconnected elements; this process can seem as overwhelming and unmanageable to the therapist as it does to the family.

Family members, though often acutely aware of the numerous obstacles they face, are less clear about how to solve them, and it is possible for the therapist to become trapped in this negative perspective as well. When one crisis is quickly followed by another, the focus becomes stuck on "putting out brush fires" as opposed to creating a powerful change. The families' existing strengths and resources become obscured in the face of the numerous obstacles. The weight of the various troubles often tips the scale and, like the family, the therapist stops trying to rebalance it.

Unfortunately, much of the training therapists receive has been in how "to map the prison, but not the escape" (Waters & Lawrence, 1993b, p. 54). Based on the traditional medical model, clinicians are educated in how to recognize and codify human pathology, with proportionately less time spent learning how to recognize clients' strengths and help them make better use of them. The depth and constancy of the problems are tracked, but thinking creatively about how to transform them is left out of the equation. Therapists need a model that provides a "path through the pathology" (Waters & Lawrence, 1993a), one that orients them to be both respectful of a family's difficulties while also holding a healthier vision for them. A competence approach (Waters & Lawrence; Lawrence & Heller, 2002) offers such a guide to this essential work with families with multiple problems.

## A COMPETENCE APPROACH DEFINED

Building on the seminal work of Robert White (1959), a developmental psychologist who studied humans' inherent striving for mastery, David Waters and Edith Lawrence (1993a) developed an innovative approach that focuses on revealing clients' underlying competence and reconnection with their inherent energy for mastery, belonging, and autonomy. White posited that all people have an innate competence motivation to master their surroundings; they want to do well and be effective at the tasks that are important to them. Infants, for example, become mesmerized as they learn a new skill—such as opening a cabinet door—and repeat the movement over and over until they feel a sense of mastery. White conceptualized this motivation less as a desire for omnipotence over someone or something than as energy spent in developing the ability to affect the world.

This resulting feeling of efficacy, gained from experiencing competence over time, develops into a confident feeling that one's presence can make a difference. Connecting to this sense of worth both produces hope and reduces the sense of powerlessness. A competence approach to therapy offers a map for seeing the interconnection between a client's health and pathology, and capitalizing on the healthy, striving energy that is fundamental to all humans (Waters & Lawrence, 1993a).

### Case Study: Susan and Her Daughter, Ellen

Susan, a young, single mother, had managed her diabetes successfully for the most part, until, for safety and financial reasons, she and her eight-year-old daughter Ellen had been forced to move in with Susan's parents. When the parents began micromanaging Susan's life, she became resentful and resistant, which made Ellen anxious and the grandparents upset. In short, all felt like failures.

The hospital psychologist was asked to consult with the family, but rather than simply tracking Susan's diabetes-management difficulties, her parents' intrusiveness, or her daughter's anxiety, she also wondered how each had become "a warrior in addition to a worrier," given the uncertainties that come with living with diabetes. This reminder of their strengths lightened the mood in the room and led to each sharing personal examples of "warrior" moments. For instance, Ellen had learned to recognize the early signs of her mother needing emergency care and could dial 911 by herself; Susan checked her glucose level on a regular basis even when she was depressed; and her parents resisted going into their daughter's bedroom every night to check on her (bringing a laugh, as no one knew they had even considered this).

As they talked, each was moved by the courage of the others, something that had been obscured in their daily battling. Energized, they were able to move away from assigning blame and toward strategizing new ways in which each might better support the warrior in all of them. A competence approach orients therapy toward recognizing and reinforcing the inherent energy of humans to master their worlds, with an eye to helping families successfully harness this force.

## UNDERLYING ASSUMPTIONS

A competence approach to therapy builds on three assumptions.

The first is that, at their core, people's motivations are healthy, and pathology an overlay to this healthy core. As White noted, infants enter life with an inherent striving to master their world, to explore and succeed at those "tasks" put before them. When guided by sensitive and responsive caregivers, their sense of competence grows; without such secure attachment figures in their life, though the desire to be competent is still there, they are less convinced of their ability to be successful, leading them to become unsure of their impact on the world.

In their approach to treating explosive, noncompliant children, Ross Greene and his colleagues (Greene, 1998; Greene & Ablon, 2006) also assume that children's inherent motivation is healthy, proposing, "children do well if they can" versus "children do well if they want to" (Greene, 2003). Their premise is that these children have "lagging skills in the global domains of flexibility/adaptability, frustration tolerance, and problem solving" (Greene & Ablon, 2006, p. 7). They suggest that a child's noncompliance is best conceptualized as a developmental delay in specific skill areas, rather than a lack of motivation to do well. Treatment focuses on accurately assessing which cognitive skills are lagging and addressing them, thereby freeing children's natural desire to do well.

Conceptualizing people's core motivations as healthy has important implications for therapy. When therapists assume pathology at the core, they may be less likely to develop a close relationship with clients for fear of discovering or unleashing more pathology. If, on the other hand, therapists assume that clients have an underlying motivation to do well, they are more likely to move toward their clients in order to better understand and connect with this healthy energy. The focus then becomes finding what in the clients' lives is constraining them from evidencing healthier behaviors, rather than fearing what other pathology might be set free by getting to know clients better. Pathology is conceptualized as just a part of who this person is—and not necessarily the most important part (Waters & Lawrence, 1993a).

Interestingly, the assumption that people are healthy at their core is one most clinicians make about themselves and those they love, even if they or their loved ones are struggling with significant problems or pathology. It only makes sense, then, to make this same assumption about our clients. Similar to the change in orientation that occurred when professionals moved away from labeling children as their problems (e.g., a learning-disabled child) and toward identifying them as having a problem (e.g., a child with a learning disability), presuming that health underlies pathology makes space for the discovery of health, even when it is not clearly visible.

The second assumption of a competence approach is that while people possess both health and pathology, these opposing functions are intertwined and the energy currently embedded in pathology can also be used for health (Waters & Lawrence, 1993a). This assumption of interconnection is based on the personality theory of Andras Angyal (1965), which postulates that humans have within them two competing systems that organize thinking and behavior—one "healthy" and the other "neurotic." When operating out of their healthy system, people view themselves and others with "loving confidence," aware of their strengths and comfortable with their limitations. When they operate out of their neurotic system, their approach to the world is one of "fearful diffidence." They are more likely to see their surroundings as hostile and cold, putting the primary focus on their own and others' limitations.

Angyal suggests that although the two systems are formed in relation to each other, if one becomes dominant, it tends to organize the total life of the person, indeed blocking the ability to see the other side. Just as it is difficult to perceive both sides of the classic figure/ground example (i.e., the picture of a vase and a woman's face), it may be difficult to see the health in people when they are operating out of their neurotic sides. Nevertheless, both sides do exist and the same experiences and feelings that fuel peoples' neurotic sides also have a link with the healthy side. Evidence for this important "both/and" rather than "either/or" connection between health and pathology is found in the power of reframing. For instance, clients often experience new energy when their anger is reframed as hurt or their defensiveness is understood as masking vulnerability. Angyal suggests "health is present potentially in its full power in the most destructive, most baneful, most shameful behavior" (1965, p. 104).

While assuming an interconnection between health and pathology can help therapists resist the pull of categorizing people as either "healthy" or "pathological," more importantly, it puts a premium on understanding the alternating relationship between both parts. Using a glass of water as a metaphor, people are neither just half full nor just half empty—they are both. The interconnection between people's health and pathology provides a richer understanding of their underlying, potentially positive energy.

For therapists working with families who have multiple problems, the successful path through the pathology comes from looking for the family's potentially healthy energy that is currently fueling problematic behavior, and redirecting it toward healthier outcomes. For example, how might a marginally employed father and his adolescent son's energy, now embedded in a battle for dominance between them, be redirected toward helping them connect with their underlying desire to feel respected by the other? Or, how might a recently divorced mother's outbursts at her children be connected to her fears that she won't be able to parent well on her own? The path through a family's multiple problems comes from understanding both their health and pathology, and most importantly, the potentially healthy striving that fuels both.

The third assumption of a competence approach is that underlying people's unhealthy behaviors are intentions for healthy behaviors. This assumption is based on Self-Determination Theory (Connell & Wellborn, 1991; Ryan & Deci, 2000), which postulates that people's behavior is motivated by one of three basic psychosocial needs—the need to feel competent, connected, and autonomous. Simply put, humans want to do well, be connected to close others, and have a say in decisions important to them. Thus, while not all behaviors are healthy, all began with a healthy intention to meet a basic need. Understanding what initially motivated the behavior (i.e., the need to feel competent, connected, and/or autonomous) can help the therapist discover clients' healthy intentions, putting the process of reconnecting to that healthy energy in motion.

As mentioned earlier, the underlying motivation to feel competent has been espoused by others (Greene & Ablon, 2006; White, 1959). The fundamental soundness of the idea that people want to do well is most apparent when juxtaposed with the opposite assumption—that they want to do a mediocre job on those things important to them. That some journeys do not turn out well does not negate the fact that the person embarked on the journey with the desire to be successful.

Similarly, attachment research has clearly established the importance of the human desire for connection with important others (Cassidy & Shaver, 1999). Several approaches to family and marital therapy have at their core the value of conceptualizing clients' problems as stemming from perceived loss of a central relationship or connection (Johnson & Whiffen, 2003). Letting clients know that their healthy need for attachment is understood and respected often frees them to be able to seek closeness and connection more successfully. And while the powerful energy behind the human need for autonomy is clearest with toddlers and adolescents, the importance of clients knowing that they have a say in the direction being taken has been well-established as a critical ingredient in successful therapy (Miller & Rollnick, 2002).

A competence approach offers a guide for conceptualizing people's behavior as being motivated by a desire to feel successful, connect with important others, and participate in making important decisions. It helps therapists look for these healthy intentions underlying unhealthy outcomes. With this as the focus, therapy shifts from blame and accusation to compassion and possibility, no matter how many problems a family has.

## TRANSLATION TO THERAPY

Waters and Lawrence (1993a; Lawrence & Heller, 2002) outline four foci that guide the use of a competence-based approach in therapy. While not formulaic, these elements can be foundational in a therapist's efforts to help families struggling with multiple problems reconnect with their underlying healthy energy and direct it toward meaningful change. The four components are: (1) understanding the client's pathology and healthy strivings; (2) developing a vision for change; (3) appreciating the courage needed for change; and (4) developing collaborative partnerships.

### 1. Understanding Pathology and Healthy Strivings

People come by their problems honestly and deserve an appreciation of the difficulties and setbacks they have experienced on their journey. A competence approach is not suggesting the therapist ignore or minimize troubles, but rather search out and understand the healthy motives and energy that are part of the behavior. According to Waters and Lawrence, too often therapists "confuse the patterns of dysfunction with the person" (1993b, p. 58). A competence approach reorients the therapist away from a fixation on deficits and dysfunction and toward identification of the competence or healthy intention presently embedded in unhealthy behavior.

### *Case Study: The Auguste Family*

The Auguste family was referred to family therapy by 12-year-old Zac's school counselor because he seemed either angry or withdrawn much of the school day. The counselor knew that Zac's six-year-old brother, Henri, was also having difficulties in school, including inattention in class and hitting other children. A single parent who recently immigrated to the United States with her sons from Haiti, Ms. Auguste was a housekeeper for the local hospital.

In the first family session, Ms. Auguste angrily shared her concerns. She was worried that Zac was "learning from bad boys" in the neighborhood: he had recently threatened to hit her when she blocked him from leaving the house after dark, later mumbling that he was going to kill Henri for breaking his radio. Henri was difficult as well; he paid little attention to what she said and she felt it time for him to "grow up." Although she shared that she tried not to physically punish the boys now, she was at a loss as to what to do when they did not listen to her. As she continued her litany of the boys' offenses, Zac withdrew and Henri began bouncing in his chair and emptying his backpack. Just as quickly as she had gotten angry with them, Ms. Auguste shut down.

As is typical for families with a multitude of concerns, their pathologies were quickly showcased. Ms. Auguste vacillated between being too harsh and feeling hopeless, and the boys ignored her as they disappeared into their own worlds. The coercive cycle (Patterson, 1982) between mother and sons was clear. Less clear was their health. Anger and sullen resistance was the pattern when they were doing poorly, but what about when they were doing well?

Sensing that the session was slipping away from her, the therapist brought out a large bag of puppets and spread them out on the floor. The mood in the room lightened as everyone grabbed for a puppet. Using the family puppet interviewing strategy outlined by Gil (1994), the therapist invited the family to work together to tell a story about their family. What emerged was a wonderful tale led by Zac that told of Dracula (his puppet) wanting to go outside, being allowed to by the Mother Shark (Ms. Auguste's puppet), but failing to come in when told, and then not being allowed to go out again. As Zac noted, "The moral of the story is if your mother lets you go out, come in on time or you can't go out again."

As revealing as the content of the puppet story was the family's sweet playfulness and care evidenced toward one another. Ms. Auguste easily joined the boys in the puppet play and was appreciative of Zac's lead. On the other hand, her difficulty understanding English became apparent as she missed Zac's insight about listening, and as the Mother Shark, she continued to scold Dracula for not minding her. This irritated Zac and he withdrew. Henri was active and not well-focused in the puppet play, but Zac was gentle, even as Henri kept hitting Zac's sore knee with his puppet; Henri's hitting seemed to come more from his desire to be included than from wanting to hurt Zac. Was this perhaps true for Henri with his peers at school as well? His healthy intention might be to be included, but he "asked" poorly. Likewise, Zac seemed to accept the need to listen to his mother, but became frustrated that she missed when he was complying. Had this also happened with his teachers at school?

The play offered an opportunity to see the family's underlying competence intertwined with their pathology. While each family member's healthy intentions were always there, it required active searching to reveal them. People have many more healthy motives than we are taught to recognize. However distorted the presentation, when we look for competence, we find it. A competence approach assumes the problems in this family were "adaptive attempts gone awry" (Waters & Lawrence, 1993a, p. 9). While Henri's hitting could be seen as a desire to be the boss, it could also be viewed as his longing to connect. Ms. Auguste's harsh parenting could be seen as a sign of her not caring or of her fear that she could not prevent Zac from turning "bad." While Zac's aggression and withdrawal from his mother may, in part, be a product of his anger about her rules, the healthier and more useful component may be his desire to succeed as a son, coupled with not knowing how and still negotiate his 12-year-old world. By empathizing with and highlighting the healthy component of Zac's anger, the therapist could help him redirect his efforts for autonomy, without jeopardizing his connection with his mother.

Though it would be easy to assume that people's inherent competence is simply the flip side of their pathology, this is not always the case. While anger sometimes masks sadness and abuse can mask caring, in order to find clients' healthy intentions, the therapist must ferret out the whole story. A competence frame with families with multiple problems helps the therapist pay special attention to underlying healthy intentions.

## 2. Developing a Vision for the Therapy

Helping people identify their vision for the future is another key element to a competence approach to therapy. Borrowing from the wisdom in *Alice's Adventures in Wonderland* (Carroll, 1865), Waters and Lawrence (1993a) note that in therapy as well as in life, "if you don't know where you're going, any road can take you there." Often families with multiple problems are so burdened with failures that they and their therapist attempt to problem-solve while still disconnected from the family's hopes and dreams for the future; in the mayhem of multiple stressors, they may reactively take the first "road" available, rather than choose one that connects with a longer-term vision. It is critical for both the therapist and family to be clear about the "big picture" (i.e., the family's dreams for the child or family) before exploring the particulars (i.e., specific goals).

Creating a vision with families can not only help to re-root the family in their own desire for something better and give them access to new energy for acting on it, it also provides a therapeutic compass. Helping families to define their vision helps keep the therapy coherent, rather than wandering from crisis to crisis. Instead of just addressing what the family is doing wrong, in a competence approach, the therapist works to help families feel safe enough to share both their hopes and their concerns, allowing both to be molded into a shared vision for the direction of change.

### *Case Study: The Howard Family*

Ms. Howard, a single mother of seven children, ages 3 to 15, was referred for in-home family therapy because her children were often late for school and left unsupervised at the housing project where they lived. The oldest ones were also beginning to become involved in delinquent activities, including shoplifting and drug use. The family had a long history of having been physically and mentally abused by Ms. Howard's former husband and had only recently been moved to this new city by child protective services to escape him.

Using a competence approach, the therapist explored with the family what they wished for their lives. Although initially cautious, everyone soon became excited about the idea of having "more fun" as a family and fighting less with one another; one of the younger children shared that she wanted to be "a joyful family for a change." In order to have more joy, the family agreed that establishing daily routines around getting ready for school, eating dinner together, and going to bed on time would help them spend less time fussing and more time enjoying life together.

Unfortunately, this new resolve to follow family rules fizzled whenever a rule (e.g., come in at dark for dinner) was applied to one of the older children. Ms. Howard could initially set a consequence, but backed down when she encountered an angry response. The more the therapist tried to put her in charge, the more the older children challenged her, leaving her in a collapsed state.

Deciding to meet Ms. Howard without the children, the therapist began by revisiting the woman's vision for her family. While she still wanted them to do well in school and fight less, she had no sense of herself as someone who could make this happen; certainly not surprising for a woman with her history of abuse, she felt powerless. Undeterred, the therapist asked her to describe her sense of a powerful woman—how she looked or what she did that made her strong. In addition to the expected answer (i.e., someone who could make her children behave or not allow herself to be abused), Ms. Howard stated that powerful women "could drive a car." Since her youth, she had thought driving a car was a sign of courage and power but had been too frightened to learn.

After developing the link between being in charge of a car and being in charge of a family, the therapist proposed teaching Ms. Howard how to drive as a first step in teaching her how to "drive" her family. For the first time in many weeks, Ms. Howard became excited and energetic about the possibility of change. With the therapist's support, she could envision herself learning to drive a car, and from this she could begin to visualize herself as powerful enough to be in charge of her children. This vision not only provided a theme for the therapy, but when broken into small steps, also helped Ms. Howard stay energized for maintaining her successes. Her children were excited about her new-found confidence and slowly learned to trust that their mother could be in charge—of a car and the family.

### 3. Appreciating the Courage Needed for Change

The third focus of a competence approach is actually taking proactive steps to help families move toward their vision. The field of mental health has failed to acknowledge how difficult it is to shift from fixed, maladaptive patterns into healthy ones. Waters and Lawrence (1993a) highlight the importance of both the clients' and therapist's courage if change is to occur. Courage is often an essential aspect of a family progressing toward their vision for change. For example, it required courage for Ms. Howard to learn to drive a car and then translate that sense of power into "driving" her family out of chaos into a situation of stability and predictability. Similarly, it required courage for the diabetic young mother and her family to hold on to their sense of themselves as "warriors" in the ongoing battle with a chronic disease, when settling into a pattern of worrying was the easier route. Change requires the courage both to recognize that a pattern of behavior is maladaptive and to risk trying something different.

A competence approach also requires courage from the therapist. Chronicling the setbacks or becoming pessimistic about the possibility of change is a temptation when working with families with multiple problems as the work is challenging and the successes often few and far between. Yet, continuing to believe in and seek out a family's healthy intentions is the key to success. Discovering the underlying health must transpire in order for clients to make use of this energy for positive outcomes. As Waters and Lawrence note, the word encourage means, literally, "to provide with courage" (1993a, p. 99).

*Case Study: Joe and Mary*

Joe and Mary's first session with a therapist who took a competence approach was a disaster. The couple had an overwhelming number of limitations and few resources for parenting their four- and two-year-old children with special needs (i.e., one had serious attention difficulties and the other had developmental delays). The children would be difficult for skilled parents to parent successfully, and Joe and Mary lacked not only the necessary expertise, but were themselves mildly retarded and had been physically abused and neglected in their own families. In the session the children ran around the office, yelling and knocking into furniture, while their parents chased behind them, shrieking threats. Halfway through the session, the therapist had mentally thrown in the towel; the only positive she could find was that a social worker from child protective services was already involved in monitoring them.

Then she stopped herself, remembering that these parents had sought out therapy precisely because they wanted to learn how to be better parents (and not lose their children). Were there other signs of competence hidden behind their very incompetent parenting? Yes. Joe had snuck in a kiss when asked to restrain the older child from climbing on the bookcase, even as the boy was kicking him, and Mary had done the same as she struggled to manage the younger one on her lap. In addition to the obvious pathology, there were signs of caring as well.

In the second session, the therapist met with the parents alone, hoping to connect more fully with the hints of underlying competencies and healthy intentions she had glimpsed in the first session. Her persistence paid off. Joe wept as he shared that he was determined to be a better father to his children than his had been to him. And while Mary was more difficult to reach, it was after all she who had insisted on coming to therapy. Although her healthy intentions were masked by her aloof and tough demeanor, the therapist wondered if her feistiness was part of the competence that held the family together. Working with the couple to help them to learn to parent in a healthy way would require a lot of work and courage on both sides; their problems were significant and resources limited. Yet, the therapist had taken the first step—searching for their underlying competence and finding the courage to believe in it.

While there may be truly impossible cases, Waters and Lawrence (1993a) hold the belief that many therapists simply do not expect enough of their clients, themselves, or therapy. When clients are confronted with setbacks or become entrenched in their dysfunction, it is easy for the therapist to become cautious, eventually losing hope as well. Uncovering and then trusting his or her courage to find a new path following a misstep challenges clients to do the same. In a competence approach to therapy, the iterative process of modeling courage for clients and finding inspiration in their courage is the foundation of success.

### 4. Build Collaborative Partnerships

The final focus of a competence approach with families with multiple problems is fundamental to all good therapy: building a collaborative partnership (Waters & Lawrence, 1993a). The therapeutic relationship is recognized as therapy's primary tool, and a competence approach builds on this premise. In order for families to feel safe enough to stretch for their dreams, the members must feel respected, even given past failures. While honoring families' pathology, taking a competence approach requires being relentless in the search for underlying healthy intentions embedded in unhealthy behavior.

Waters and Lawrence (1993a) emphasize that key to this search is for the therapist to look for and discover what he or she loves about the family. In the process of this discovery they will also uncover the family's healthy intentions. As importantly, clients are often empowered by the therapist's belief that there is more to them than their maladaptive and often irritating traits, and they begin to strive more strongly for change. A useful reminder is the saying, "People don't care how much you know until they know how much you care." Adopting a nonhierarchical, nonblaming stance in therapy allows room for mistakes to be redefined as adaptive attempts gone awry. This collaborative, interpersonal process can inspire both therapist and client to access the strength required to make change viable.

## CONCLUSION

At its core, a competence approach is about bringing out the best in families and helping them reconnect with their desires for mastery, belonging, and autonomy that have become obscured by maladaptive patterns. The desire to be successful is universal, however distorted the presentation. Search for dysfunction, we will find it. Search for health, we will find it as well. A competence approach offers a map for locating the interconnection between health and pathology, and organizes therapy around the underlying healthy striving. Acknowledging and valuing the competencies of families wrestling with multiple problems magnifies the possibility that they will learn to lead with their best.

## REFERENCES


Angyal, A. (1965). *Neurosis and treatment: A holistic theory*. New York: Wiley.

Cassidy, J. & Shaver, P. (1999). *Handbook of attachment: Theory, research and clinical applications*. New York: Guilford Press.

Carroll, L. (1865). *Alice's adventures in wonderland*. England: Macmillan.

Connell, J. P., & Wellborn, J. G. (1991). Competence, autonomy, and relatedness: A motivational analysis of self-system processes. In R. Gunnar & L. A. Sroufe (Eds.), *Minnesota symposia on child psychology* (Vol. 23, pp. 43–77). Hillsdale, NJ: Lawrence Erlbaum Associates.

Gil, E. (1994). *Play in family therapy*. New York: Guilford Press.

Greene, R. W. (1998). *The explosive child*. New York: Harper Collins.

Greene, R. W. (2003, November). *Collaborative approaches with explosive children and adolescents*. Keynote presented at the Astor Home Annual Mental Health Conference, Rhinebeck, NY.

Greene, R. W., & Ablon, J. S. (2006). *Treating explosive kids: The collaborative problem-solving approach*. New York: Guilford Press.

Johnson, S. M., & Whiffen, V. (2003). *Attachment processes in couples and families*. New York: Guilford Press.

Lawrence, E. C., & Heller, M. C. (2002). Parent-school collaboration: The utility of a competence approach. *Canadian Journal of School Psychology, 17*, 5–15.

Miller, W. R., & Rollnick, S. (2002). *Motivational interviewing: Preparing people for change*. New York: Guilford Press.

Patterson, G. R. (1982). *Coercive family process*. Eugene, OR: Castalia.

Ryan, R. M., & Deci, E. L. (2000). Self-determination theory and the facilitation of intrinsic motivation, social development, and well-being. *American Psychologist, 55*, 68–78.

Stormshak, E. A., & Dishion, T. J. (2002). An ecological approach to child and family clinical and counseling psychology. *Clinical Child and Family Psychology Review, 5*(3), 197–215.

Waters, D., & Lawrence, E. (1993a). *Competence, courage, and change: An approach to family therapy*. New York: W. W. Norton & Company.

Waters, D., & Lawrence, E. (1993b). Creating a therapeutic vision. *Family Therapy Networker, 17*, 52–58.

White, R. W. (1959). Motivation reconsidered: The concept of competence. *Psychological Review, 66*, 297–333.

# 11

# Strengths-Based Approaches with Adolescents and Families of Color

*Jennifer Lee*

A strengths-based approach with families is a particular perspective that sees families as inherently resilient. This approach challenges the idea of a "dysfunctional family," a term so commonplace in our lexicon that we may not know what it means to be a "functional family." Rather than seeing families as repositories for our failings, we can honor families for challenging our capacities and reaffirming our connections with one another (DeFraine & Asay, 2007). With a strengths-based perspective, we recognize the multitude of strengths that families bring with them into the therapy room. Culture and ethnicity is one such area of strength.

Smith (2006a) points out that an essential component of strengths-based therapy is the understanding that culture has a significant impact on how individuals consider and evaluate human strengths. She explains that each individual's greatest area of potential growth resides within his or her strengths. Identifying a person's cultural strengths is one way to build on his or her preexisting competencies.

This chapter focuses on strengths-based therapy with adolescents and families of color. This perspective integrates core multicultural competencies as described by Sue, Arredondo, and McDavis (1992), including the therapist's awareness of his or her own culture, knowledge of the worldview of the culturally different client, and the use of culturally appropriate treatment interventions. The main distinction of the strengths-based approach, however, is the focused search for cultural strengths in an effort to build confidence, foster empowerment, promote shared understanding, and increase commitment to therapy.

## ADOPTING A STRENGTHS-BASED PERSPECTIVE

As therapists, we may be privileged with clinical moments full of meaning and insight that continue to guide our work long after termination. I'd like to share one such moment that helped me experientially understand the power of a strengths-based perspective.

I had the opportunity to work with "Andrea" while training on an inpatient unit of a large city hospital. She brought herself to the emergency room reportedly feeling unsafe after hearing voices in her apartment that were threatening to hurt her. Andrea was an African American woman in her mid-30s. She had a successful career as an artist, but her long-term plans changed in her late 20s when the first signs of mental illness became evident. Over the years, Andrea grew to recognize the warning signs of her illness and would voluntarily bring herself to the hospital and stay at the inpatient unit until her condition stabilized. Afterwards, she was able to return home to an independent life.

Upon admission to the unit, I worked with Andrea providing supportive therapy while the attending psychiatrist closely monitored her medications. During our first encounters, Andrea was reserved and somewhat withdrawn. Some days, Andrea agreed to meet with me for a while, but other times, she grew tired after a few minutes and asked that she be left alone. During the initial period of her hospitalization, doubts about the usefulness of my role as a therapist surfaced. I wondered how I could possibly help her. Given her diagnosis, wasn't it more important that she comply with her medication regime?

Andrea's acute psychotic symptoms gradually dissipated the longer she spent on the unit. During this time, Andrea became more engaged in our sessions and began to openly share personal aspects of her life. She wove together a rich history of her early career as an artist, the influences of her cultural background as an African American woman, her spiritual and religious identity as a Christian, and her extended family who came to visit her regularly at the hospital. During our sessions, she guided me along this personal journey beyond the boundaries of her mental illness. As she felt safer in the therapeutic setting, she began to look forward to our sessions and quietly expressed her gratitude for the opportunity to share her life in this way.

It slowly became apparent to me that I had been asking the wrong question all along. I wondered how I could possibly help Andrea given the complexity of her diagnosis and her need for long-term medications. I was looking at this case with a medical-model mind-set, through the static lens of pathology. During one session, Andrea shared an insight that became a transformative experience for both of us. In that moment, Andrea became my greatest teacher.

Andrea spent the morning working out with a trainer in the unit's weight room. She talked to her trainer about wanting to lose the extra weight she had put on recently while at the hospital. The trainer instructed, "Don't focus on what you don't want. Focus on what you want." Andrea explained to me in session, "So instead of telling myself, I *don't want* a big belly or I *don't want* flabby arms, I can say, I *want* a strong body and I *want* a healthy lifestyle." In her revelatory moment, she understood that she didn't have to continue focusing on what was going wrong in her life. Instead, she could focus on what she wanted and capitalize on the strengths she already possessed. She had come to accept the realities of her condition and the necessity of complying with her medication regime. She, however, was not defined or confined by the limitations of her illness. She experienced much success in early adulthood, and she was motivated to continue her work in the arts with the support of her family and friends. As she prepared herself for discharge, she excitedly discussed her plans to continue working and contributing to her art community with a steadfast determination to cultivate a meaningful life.

In our last sessions together, Andrea spoke about her spiritual and religious beliefs. Although she strongly identified with her Christian faith, she had a growing interest in Eastern religions and spiritual teachings. She referred to His Holiness the Dalai Lama, who said, "Be kind whenever possible. It is always possible." Andrea was struck by the poetry of the word "possible." She said, "The Dalai Lama didn't say, 'always be kind.' Instead, he said that being kind is always possible, meaning that it's a choice. We can choose to be kind because it's always available to us." Andrea sat silently for a moment, to absorb the meaning of her interpretation. She looked at me and quietly reiterated, "It's a choice."

Andrea, in her moments of insight, gave me my own. In the years since I've thanked Andrea over and over in my mind for giving me this priceless gift. The shift in perspective, from a pathology-focused mind-set to a strengths-based one, is subtle. Yet, as Andrea intuited, it's a choice. We can choose to focus on what's wrong with our clients and work on their weaknesses, or we can choose to highlight areas of strength and harness their innate capacities toward healing and growth. With this mind-set, we can connect with our clients in a humanistic way that transcends labels and diagnoses, and honors the resilience of the human spirit.

## CHALLENGES IN THERAPY WITH YOUTH AND FAMILIES OF COLOR

In the recent past, multiculturalism has been identified as the "fourth force" in counseling, following the movements of psychodynamic, behavioral, and humanistic psychology (Essandoh, 1996; Pedersen, 1999). Multiculturalism encompasses race, ethnicity, and culture, as well as age, gender, social class, sexual orientation, physical ability, and religious identity. While this movement has prompted counselors to consider the multiple sociocultural factors that impact the therapeutic process and relationship, specific challenges arise when working with culturally diverse youth and families. For one, people of color continue to face significant barriers to treatment. Secondly, the counseling framework of multiculturalism presents challenges for therapists as evident in the current discourse in cross-cultural psychology.

### Barriers to Treatment

As a group, people of color may be less likely to utilize counseling services because seeking help outside the family would be considered a violation of cultural norms. Among Asian cultures, for example, "saving face" is a strong cultural deterrent for individuals in need of mental health treatment. A label of mental illness carries serious social stigma, which can bring humiliation and shame, and damage the reputation of the family (Chen & Swartzman, 2001).

Cultural expectations around emotional expressiveness present another barrier to treatment. Whereas individuals in Western cultures may be accustomed to talking about their feelings in the service of emotional catharsis, Eastern cultures emphasize the control and suppression of emotions as an adaptive coping strategy (Chen & Swartzman, 2001). In this manner, self-restraint is a culturally sanctioned attribute where individuals are expected to behave in a way that maintains the harmony and stability of social relationships for the benefit of group functioning. Since Western forms of psychotherapy rely on the individual's ability to verbalize his or her affective experiences, expressing feelings may feel disgraceful for Asian clients who are expected to demonstrate emotional restraint.

Other barriers to treatment for youth and families of color include lack of awareness of the available services in the community and a reluctance to seek help based on previous experiences of discrimination from social service agencies (Vera & Shin, 2006). Latinos in the United States with uncertain immigration status face special challenges, and may not take advantage of educational, social, and health care assistance for fears of deportation, arrest, or job loss (de Leon Siantz, 1997).

### Universalism versus Relativism

An ongoing debate in cross-cultural psychology exists between the seemingly opposing perspectives of cultural universalism and cultural relativity.

Generally speaking, universalistic (etic) approaches search for common strengths while relativistic (emic) approaches focus on ethnic-specific strengths (Berry, Poortinga, Segall, & Dasen, 1992). For the study of family life, the universalistic perspective embraces a comparative search for cross-cultural similarities, and assumes that family relationships have stable and constant patterns across social groups. In contrast, the relativistic perspective considers indigenous relationship patterns that are distinctive of a particular culture (Peterson, 2007).

Gary Peterson (2007) asserts that these perspectives are complementary processes that enrich one another, and encourages their integration in the examination of family strengths to enhance cross-cultural understanding. He explains that an effort to categorize such approaches as oppositional builds "false dichotomies" that fail to capture the rich complexities that exist in social life. While universals exist, "cultural diversity within family strengths is likely to be found in the details that are nestled within broader commonalities" (p. xxviii). J. W. Berry (1999) also refutes the notion that emic and etic approaches pose a dilemma in a tension of antagonistic forces. He recognizes their symbiotic relationship and views each perspective as different points of entry in understanding human behavior.

Wei Zhang (2006) offers one way to transcend opposing viewpoints, and sees cross-cultural understanding as a hermeneutic riddle rather than a problem to be solved or pieces of a puzzle to fit together. The riddle is likened to a Zen koan—a seemingly paradoxical story, question, or statement that cannot be solved by logical explanation or rational interpretation. Zhang writes, "The koan constantly engages the listeners who are listening to its moral message; as each time it speaks, it speaks anew" (p. 7). This perspective is offered as one step toward enhancing and promoting cross-cultural understanding. But first, we must be willing to listen.

Smith (2006a) further points out that the central construct of oppression has been a point of emphasis in the multicultural counseling literature, rather than the meaningful contact that people of color share. She encourages cross-cultural counselors to focus on clients' cultural and individual strengths, rather than "the victimization effects of racial or ethnic discrimination" (p. 17). An identification of cultural strengths allows clients to build on these existing competencies that have allowed them to survive and grow.

With the current discourse in mind, a strengths-based approach can appear to transcend the dichotomy between universalism and relativism, and the mutually exclusive labels of victim and oppressor. The therapist who embraces a strengths-based approach is suspended in a space beyond concepts, labels, and socially constructed dualities, yet connected to his or her client through shared language and understanding.

## REFRAMING CHALLENGES AND HARNESSING STRENGTHS

Strengths-based interventions have been fundamental to the field of family therapy since its beginnings. Reframing is a basic tenet of family therapy in which an experience previously considered negative is recontextualized as something positive or functional (Watzlawick, Weakland, & Fisch, 1974). Using a different perceptual lens, the act of reframing changes the entire meaning of an experience.

In recent decades, the field of family therapy has evolved with new theoretical approaches predominantly centered on clients' strengths. In narrative approaches, families learn to tell their life stories from a strengths-based position, and in doing so, change the meaning they have attributed to negative life events that are stressful, painful, and traumatic (White & Epston, 1990). Smith (2006a) understands that helping our clients make meaning of their circumstances and shifting the viewpoint from seeing oneself as a survivor instead of a victim can have a powerful effect during therapy. Through empowerment, clients understand that they have a choice in how they perceive adversities or hardships, and they can play an active role in deconstructing unproductive stories in order to reconstruct new ones (Nichols, 2008). Similarly, solution-focused approaches embrace the basic assumptions that people are inherently resilient and resourceful (de Shazer et al., 2007). It helps clients learn to speak the prospective, positive language of solutions rather than the past-focused, negative language of problems.

A strengths-based approach can traverse different theoretical orientations by shifting the focus from problems to solutions, from challenges to strengths. For families of color, it also requires honoring relevant cultural strengths such as ethnic identity, bicultural identity, strong kinship network, and spiritual or religious identity (Harrison-Hale, McLoyd, & Smedley, 2004; Vera & Shin, 2006; Villalba, 2007).

### Ethnic Identity

The development of a healthy ethnic identity is an essential strategy for building strength and resiliency in youth of color (Querimit & Conner, 2003; Vera & Shin, 2006), and serves an important function in providing adolescents with a sense of safety, self-esteem, and belonging (Smith, 2006b).

According to Smith (2006b), a strengths-based approach to therapy underscores the positive impact of communities with a strong collective identity and ties among its members. This sense of community can serve a protective function for youth against the toxic influences of the environment such as drug abuse and violence. Smith explains, "We tend to feel strong when we have a clear sense of who we are and how we fit into the world. We feel our strength when we feel secure in the love of those surrounding us and when others support the way we think and believe" (p. 141).

Phillip Bowman (2006) also suggests that cultural strengths can help individuals maintain hope and achieve against overwhelming odds, buffering the adolescent from toxins in the social environment. For example, to help their children face the realities of racism and prejudice; some parents will foster the strengthening of identity through ethnic socialization efforts (Phinney & Chavira, 1995). Ethnic and cultural socialization may protect youth from the deleterious effects of an environment fueled by racial discrimination, while simultaneously promoting the development of individual resiliency and self-esteem (Smith, 2006a).

## Bicultural Identity

Similar to ethnic identity, an adolescent's bicultural identity can be a significant source of strength. Being bicultural, for many youth of color, is an ongoing tension where they must navigate two worlds—one of their parents and another of their peers. There is an inherent difficulty in simultaneously understanding and being accepted by both cultures (Phinney, Cantu, & Kurtz, 1997), and these youth may feel caught straddling the divide between two distinctly different and seemingly incompatible cultures. Most adolescents may view this tension as a disadvantage, an added dimension to the already stressful developmental process of separation and individuation. Although they may be moving farther away from the old world of their parents and becoming further embedded with their peer group, youth of color maintain ties with their culture even in their newly found independence. This multifaceted challenge of living and balancing two cultures, while negotiating the demands of adolescence, is respectable and commendable because it demonstrates resilience (Villalba, 2007). A strengths-based perspective can help youth of color harness the advantages of their bicultural identity, highlighting their expanded and unique worldview, and focusing on their intrinsic strengths that have allowed them to successfully negotiate two culturally different worlds.

## Strong Kinship Network

Close ties with family and extended kin are an important source of strength for many families of color (Harrison-Hale et al., 2004; Vera & Shin, 2006). For generations, strong kinship networks have characterized African American families (Hines & Boyd-Franklin, 2005). These networks are composed of immediate and extended family members such as grandparents, aunts, uncles, and cousins, as well as nonblood relatives such as godparents, neighbors, friends, and members of the church. African American youth may consider extended family members as significant sources of support, intimacy, and companionship. Similarly, among Latino people, familismo (familialism) is an important cultural value, which involves a strong attachment and identification to immediate and extended family members (Santiago-Rivera, 2003). In this family network, compadres (godparents) play an essential role in the child's life as "coparents" who help raise and nurture the child. When working with families of color, therapists can recognize and honor the presence of important members within this network of strong family ties.

## Spirituality and Religion

Another strength for many adolescents and families of color is in the area of spirituality and religion (Vera & Shin, 2006). Dara Querimit and Latoya Conner (2003) highlight the necessity of incorporating cultural values that provide support and a higher purpose, such as spirituality, to promote healthy development among youth of color.

According to one perspective, religion has been conceptualized as a type of adaptive coping mechanism for people of color, which enables them to rise above the limitations and harsh realities of their social circumstances (Harrison-Hale et al., 2004). Religion, in this view, can help people of color adjust to their environments and provide meaning to their existence, both in the individual and collective sense.

Froma Walsh (2008) points out that most spiritual traditions worldwide, in contrast to the individualism of American culture, consider human experience as deeply embedded within the family and the surrounding community. This is true for many ethnic minority communities, where churches offer individual and community support, both spiritually and socially. For example, African American churches are important institutions for influencing belief systems and social attitudes (Harrison-Hale et al., 2004). Like most cultures with a collectivist worldview, bonds within the religious or spiritual community play a significant role in family life. Similarly, Korean ethnic churches serve important social functions including the provision of fellowship, a sense of belonging, and a place to maintain cultural traditions (Min, 1992). In one study, Korean American adolescents viewed their church youth group as a cultural sanctuary where they found comfort and solace among their extended church family (Lee, Chang, & Miller, 2006). Especially for minority youth who may encounter racism and discrimination in the school environment, the youth group serves as a safe haven where cultural traditions are acknowledged and celebrated, rather than scrutinized and ridiculed. The strengths-based approach respects spiritual and religious communities that may play a critical role in the lives of youth and families of color.

## ADVANTAGES OF A STRENGTHS-BASED MIND-SET

There are several important advantages of adopting a strengths-based mind-set with adolescents and families of color, such as empowerment, shared understanding, and increased commitment to treatment.

### Empowerment

Recognition of our clients' strengths can build motivation, confidence, and empowerment within the individual (Smith, 2006b). When clients harness their strengths, they learn that positive experiences are possible and they can play a part in engineering their own lives. While we may not have control over what happens in our lives, we have control over how we perceive and respond to these events. For adolescents and families of color, developing feelings of empowerment can help buffer the negative effects of their social environment.

### Shared Understanding

When therapists convey an openness to the strengths of clients, a sense of understanding and shared meaning between clients and therapists can emerge (Santiago-Rivera, 2003). Different worldviews among therapist and client can create schisms in the therapeutic relationship based on an inherent discrepancy in values. Using the theoretical framework of Hazel Rose Markus and Shinobu Kitayama (1991), a therapist with an individualistic worldview may prize autonomy and independence, while a client with a collectivistic orientation may value social connectedness and interdependence. When therapists and clients look through the same lens to identify and emphasize strengths, they begin to speak the same language and build meaningful connections across different worldviews.

### Increased Commitment to Therapy

Identifying clients' strengths as a therapeutic intervention enhances the therapeutic alliance and increases their motivation to invest themselves in therapy (Smith, 2006b). Considering the historic and current trends of underutilized mental health services and high drop-out rates among ethnic minority clients and families, a substantial gap exists between their unfulfilled needs and therapists' abilities to provide for their needs (Ho, Rasheed, & Rasheed, 2003). Given the preexisting barriers to treatment for culturally different youth and families, approaching therapy with the clients' strengths in mind can lower the obstacles that preclude individuals from entering treatment.

## CASE STUDY

I met "Jonathan," a 16-year-old Latino, when he presented to treatment upon the insistence of his father, "Carlos." On the intake form, Carlos indicated numerous problems in his son including lack of motivation, academic difficulties, dishonesty, and disobedience. He explained that his son was in need of individual therapy and various psychological assessments to figure out what was "wrong" with him. After gathering more information, it appeared that Jonathan was the symptom bearer of the system and a referral for family therapy was made.

Carlos was a university professor in his home country in South America, and the family lived a middle-class lifestyle. The family immigrated to the United States after Jonathan's mother died a few years earlier. Carlos explained that most of his family was in the United States, and he needed the support of his extended family because the stress of being a single father became too overwhelming. The main motivator, however, was to provide a better life for his son, which meant a better education and more job opportunities. Carlos, however, was unable to transfer his professional skills in the American education system and was required to find work in the business sector as an hourly employee for a moving company.

Jonathan was a quiet, well-mannered young man with a gentle disposition. In family sessions, he remained mostly quiet and deferential as his father lectured him about his poor academic performance and disobedient behavior. In sparse moments, Jonathan was able to express that his father was strict, overprotective, and overly demanding with his academics. Jonathan explained that his father constantly interrogated him, policed his every move, and never granted him an ounce of privacy. He admitted that it was sometimes easier to tell a white lie, rather than get the third degree from his father.

In family sessions, Carlos was very vocal about his expectations for his son, both behaviorally and academically. He felt that his son had great potential to excel in school, but saw him as "lazy and unmotivated." Carlos often grounded his son and expected him to study during every waking hour, which only created more resistance in Jonathan.

The family was negotiating several major life transitions including acculturative stress, adolescence, single parenthood, and the untimely death of

Jonathan's mother. In Carlos, I saw many generations of immigrants who came to America in search of a better life for their children. I saw my own relatives who did everything they could in the name of their children. Sacrifice is a familiar word that echoes throughout the generations. In Jonathan, I saw many children of immigrants who faced the challenge of living in two worlds. I saw myself as a teenager feeling the intense academic pressure imposed by my parents and the heavy burden of achievement. Disappointment is a common feeling passed down through the generations.

Although it was easy to remain fixated on the presenting problem that originally brought Carlos and Jonathan in for treatment, a strengths-based lens helped reframe family challenges as cultural assets. José Villalba Jr. (2007) highlights culture-specific virtues for Latino youth, such as being bilingual, being bicultural, and the strength of the family bond. Few Latino youth are aware of the advantages of being fluent in both Spanish and English, and most may not realize the marketability of their skills. For Jonathan, this meant helping him recognize his competencies, successfully living in two cultures and being fluent in two languages. Magnifying Jonathan's assets in this way aspired to bolster his self-esteem and raise his expectations for future career plans after high school and beyond.

For both father and son, a strengths-based perspective helped reframe their difficulties in the context of their close family bond. Carlos's tendency toward overprotection was understood in light of his dual responsibilities, taking on the role of both mother and father for Jonathan. Aspects of therapy then focused on helping Carlos activate the strengths of his extended family and pull in more resources to lessen his role strain as a single parent. For Jonathan, he was deep in the throes of adolescence, negotiating the tension between separation and closeness, at times wanting independence and at other times needing connection with his father. Jonathan would be graduating from high school soon but he was unable to verbalize plans for college. It became clear that he was apprehensive about going away because it meant being separated from his father. His "lack of motivation" was understood in the context of the strain born out of his protective feelings for his father.

In one family session, Carlos was able to create an authentic connection with his son, communicating with him through love rather than disappointment. He talked openly about his relationship with his own father, and how he tried to assert his independence under his father's authoritarian grip. In his playful, humorous manner, he shared a story when he attempted to sneak out of the house on one occasion and the cat-and-mouse caper that quickly ensued. Carlos brought his son back in time to when he himself was 16, a time when he was searching for his own identity and attempting to assert his autonomy. Jonathan listened intently, joining with his father in this quietly amusing and poignant moment. When his father finished his story, Jonathan looked at him and said, "Dad, I never knew what you were like at my age. Thank you for sharing that with me." Carlos replied, his eyes moist with tears, "I wanted you to know that I understand your struggle. Sometimes, though, I forget."

Virginia Satir, in *A Family at a Point of Growth* (Slayton & Gilmore, 1983), described the love shared between a father and son as a peak experience. Everyone in that room, in that moment, witnessed the power of that peak experience. Jonathan saw his father's difficulties through a multigenerational perspective, and was able to connect to the 16-year-old boy in his father who also struggled for independence. Carlos was able to empathize with his son's need for autonomy while honoring the memory of his own father. Working in the framework of strengths, father and son were able to adopt a different language which allowed them to reach one another through love and the power of their family bond.

## CONCLUSION

By solely focusing on our clients' problems and failings, we lose the opportunity to consider the qualities and aspects that have allowed them to survive. When we peer through one lens of the binocular, our vision is restricted. When we open our eyes and look through both lenses, a fuller, richer perspective is revealed. We don't ignore the problems that originally brought our families into treatment, but we don't remain fixated on them through a single lens.

When we consider the strengths inherent in the lives of our adolescents and families of color, the limitations in cross-cultural dialogue between universalism and relativism fade into the background. The cultural strengths of our clients—drawn from their ethnic identity, bonds within the family network, and ties to religious or spiritual communities—materialize into the foreground. We emphasize these aspects of experience to harness the strengths that already reside within. With this new viewpoint comes greater depth perception and broader peripheral vision. With this new perspective, we develop a shared understanding, honoring the innate capacities in our clients that have allowed them to survive, heal, and grow.

## REFERENCES

Berry, J. W. (1999). Emics and etics: A symbiotic conception. *Culture & Psychology, 5*, 165–171.

Berry, J. W., Poortinga, Y. H., Segall, M. H., & Dasen, P. R. (1992). *Cross-cultural psychology: Research and applications*. New York: Cambridge University Press.

Bowman, P. J. (2006). Role strain and adaptation issues in the strength-based model: Diversity, multilevel, and life-span considerations. *The Counseling Psychologist, 34*, 118–133.

Chen, X., & Swartzman, L. C. (2001). Health beliefs and experiences in Asian cultures. In S. S. Kazarian & D. R. Evans (Eds.), *Handbook of cultural health psychology* (pp. 389–410). San Diego, CA: Academic Press.

DeFraine, J., & Asay, S. M. (2007). Strong families around the world: An introduction to a family strengths perspective. *Marriage & Family Review, 41*, 1–10.

de Leon Siantz, M. K. (1997). Factors that impact development outcomes of immigrant children. In A. Booth, A. Crouter, & N. Landale (Eds.), *Immigration and the family: Research and policy on U.S. immigrants* (pp. 149–161). Mahwah, NJ: Erlbaum.

de Shazer, S., Dolan, Y., Korman, H., Trepper, T., Berg, I. K., & McCollum, E. (2007). *More than miracles: The state of the art of solution-focused brief therapy*. Binghamton, NY: Haworth Press.

Essandoh, P. K. (1996). Multicultural counseling as the "fourth force": A call to arms. *The Counseling Psychologist, 24*, 126–137.

Harrison-Hale, A. O., McLoyd, V., & Smedley, B. (2004). Racial and ethnic status: Risk and protective processes among African American families. In K. I. Maton, C. J. Schellenbach, B. J. Leadbeater, & A. L. Solarz (Eds.), *Investing in children, youth, families, and communities: Strengths-based research and policy* (pp. 269–283). Washington, DC: American Psychological Association.

Hines, P. M., & Boyd-Franklin, N. (2005). African American families. In M. McGoldrick, J. Giordano, & N. Garcia-Preto (Eds.), *Ethnicity and family therapy* (3rd ed., pp. 87–100). New York: Guilford Press.

Ho, M. K., Rasheed, J. M., & Rasheed, M. N. (2003). *Family therapy with ethnic minorities* (2nd ed.). Thousand Oaks, CA: Sage Publications.

Lee, J., Chang, E. S., & Miller, L. (2006). Ethnic-religious status and identity formation: A qualitative study of Korean American Christian youth. *Journal of Youth Ministry, 5*, 9–40.

Markus, H. R., & Kitayama, S. (1991). Culture and the self: implications for cognition, emotion, and motivation. *Psychological Review, 98*, 224–253.

Min, P. G. (1992). The structure and social functions of Korean immigrant churches in the United States. *International Migration Review, 26*, 1370–1394.

Nichols, M. P. (2008). *Family therapy: Concepts and methods* (8th ed.). Boston: Allyn & Bacon.

Pedersen, P. (1999). *Multiculturalism as a fourth force*. Philadelphia: Brunner/Mazel.

Peterson, G. W. (2007). Preface: Family strengths from a cross-cultural and theoretical perspective. *Marriage & Family Review, 41*, xxv–xxix.

Phinney, J. S., Cantu, C. L., & Kurtz, D. A. (1997). Ethnic and American identity as predictors of self-esteem among African American, Latino, and White adolescents. *Journal of Youth and Adolescence, 26*, 165–185.

Phinney, J. S., & Chavira, V. (1995). Parental ethnic socialization and adolescent coping with problems related to ethnicity. *Journal of Research on Adolescence, 5*, 31–53.

Querimit, D. S., & Conner, L. C. (2003). Empowerment psychotherapy with adolescent females of color. *Journal of Clinical Psychology, 59*, 1215–1224.

Santiago-Rivera, A. (2003, February). Latinos values and family transitions: Practical considerations for counseling. *Counseling and Human Development*. Retrieved March 20, 2009, from http://findarticles.com/p/articles/mi_qa3934/is_200302/ai_n9198342

Slayton, C., & Gilmore, D. (Producers). (1983). A family at the point of growth [Videorecording]. Kansas City, MO: Golden Triad Films, Inc.

Smith, E. J. (2006a). The strength-based counseling model. *The Counseling Psychologist, 34*, 13–79.

Smith, E. J. (2006b). The strength-based counseling model: A paradigm shift in psychology. *The Counseling Psychologist, 34*, 134–144.

Sue, D. W., Arredondo, P., & McDavis, R. J. (1992). Multicultural counseling competencies and standards: A call to the profession. *Journal of Multicultural Counseling and Development, 20*, 64–88.

Vera, E. M., & Shin, R. Q. (2006). Promoting strengths in a socially toxic world: Supporting resilience with systemic interventions. *The Counseling Psychologist, 34*, 80–89.

Villalba, J. A. (2007). Culture-specific assets to consider when counseling Latina/o children and adolescents. *Journal of Multicultural Counseling and Development, 35*, 15–25.

Walsh, F. (2008). Spirituality, healing, and resilience. In M. McGoldrick & K. V. Hardy (Eds.), *Re-visioning family therapy: Race, culture, and gender in clinical practice* (2nd ed., pp. 61–75). New York: Guilford Press.

Watzlawick, P., Weakland, J., & Fisch, R. (1974). *Change: Principles of problem formation and problem resolution*. New York: Norton.

White, M., & Epston, D. (1990). *Narrative means to therapeutic ends*. New York: Norton.

Zhang, W. (2006). *Heidegger, Rorty, and the Eastern thinkers: A hermeneutics of cross-cultural understanding*. Albany, NY: State University of New York Press.

# 12

# What Survivors of Military Families, 9/11, and Hurricane Katrina Teach Us about Resilience in the Wake of Trauma

*Misty Solt*

"How do you do what you do?" is the question I (and other therapists) receive quite frequently from individuals outside the counseling field in regard to working with children who've experienced trauma and grief. In attempting to question, I am cognizant of just how limited human beings are by the sole means of verbal expression. Words inadequately convey what it is like to walk with a client through the aftermath of a permanently life-altering event—an event that has turned every ounce of that person's lived predictability into pounds of loss, confusion, and change—and yet experience the indelible strength and fortitude of such individuals. As I have worked for over a decade and continue to work with individuals who have experienced such life-changing events, I am confronted daily with the fact that it can be the most painful, helpless, confusing, and fearful situations that bring to the surface the strength, courage, and determination of humankind. This can especially be seen in working with children.

Teaching and supervising master's-level graduates in the counseling program at Southern Methodist University in Plano, Texas, reminds me daily of the strong scientific focus that is needed to ultimately optimize the practice of a mental health professional. The heavy emphasis on diagnosing, theoretical adherence, skill implementation, empirical research, ethical considerations, and legal ramifications are no doubt paramount in succeeding as a mental health clinician. And yet, sitting across the room from a five-year-old child struggling to cope with the death of his mother and sister from a recent head-on vehicular collision (i.e., as well as learning to cope with his own acquired permanent injuries) brings into my awareness how reductionistic we can be while operating in the scientific mode. It only takes a moment of being with that five-year-old client to realize how essential the "art" of counseling also is. It is through the "art" of counseling that the working alliance is established, which is essential for the healing process to begin. David Crenshaw (2008) poignantly discussed this point by stating the following:

> Psychotherapy at its best is part science and part art, and I hope it always remains so. Science and empirical research inform and guide clinical practice but when the child, teen, or family enters the office or therapy room, what takes place is a unique human encounter that is as much art as science. (p. 1)

For the sake of illustrating the "art" in counseling individuals who've experience trauma and loss, I've decided to include some of the transformative experiences whose catalytic nature has impacted my embracing of a strengths-based, humanistic approach in using play therapy to work with children. Consequently, the following narratives included in this chapter are written out of a high sense of veneration for the children and families I have worked with who have experienced unusually difficult circumstances (i.e., War in Iraq, the 9/11 terrorist attacks, and Hurricane Katrina). In these anecdotes, names and other identifiable details have been altered or expunged for the protection of protected health information in compliance with HIPAA ordinances. In working with these children and families, I have learned so much about therapy, trauma, and living in general. I share these heroic examples of courage with you out of my deepest reverence for these children who have trusted me to be a part of their reconstruction of self, ego, and world in the midst of profound loss.

## CREATING A HEALING DISTANCE THROUGH THE USE OF PLAY

To begin, it is important to give an overview of three constructs important in working with children who've experienced trauma or loss: (1) play therapy is a developmentally appropriate therapeutic modality used to facilitate the expression of children; (2) through play, children often create a safe distance from the trauma as a way of initially coping; and (3) predictability (i.e., routine, consistency, etc.) is essential in engendering a sense of safety for children during such vulnerable times. Additionally, the importance of receiving proper training and supervision in working in the area of trauma and loss needs to be emphasized in order to obviate both retraumatizing effects on the child and vicarious traumatism of the clinician.

In working with children who've experienced trauma or loss, play therapy can facilitate the expression of children who are still operating in the preoperational and concrete operational phase of cognitive development. Garry

Landreth (2002) discussed that play is a child's developmentally appropriate way of expressing and processing the world at large (i.e., play being a child's language and toys being representative of words ensconced in that language). According to Landreth, children are able to employ developmentally appropriate coping mechanisms through play, which allows for the creation of a safe buffer during extreme emotional vulnerability. Furthermore, Lenore Terr (1994) maintained that sometimes children use a powerful and common developmental defense of denying in fantasy what had occurred in reality for the use of momentarily coping with a traumatic event. As an example, Terr described how children who had witnessed the 1986 Challenger explosion had recreated the disastrous outcome (i.e., the shuttle exploding) through fantasy play into a productive outcome, such as the shuttle landing safely somewhere. Bonnie Badenoch (2008) discussed that by engaging in this symbolic play (e.g., also referred to as compensatory or projective play), children are able to create a safe and healing distance from their difficult experiences. According to Badenoch, coupling this repeated symbolic play with the existence of a safe and warm therapeutic relationship, children are able to alleviate and repair the emotional pain and fear at a deeper, internal level—freeing more internal resources for the child to access for ultimate coping. Badenoch further espoused, "This repeated repair experience builds neural connections that may help related experiences become more emotionally manageable, even if children's day-to-day worlds aren't changing much" (p. 306). Additionally, play affords children who've experienced a significant change in their perceived safety some predictability by which they are able to exert control over a very out-of-control situation.

## PREDICTABILITY AS THE FORERUNNER TO SAFETY

Predictability in daily life gives a fundamental level of security needed to feel safe and to function most optimally in our environment (Landreth, 2002). Individuals, families, and cultures implement varying levels of predictability (i.e., ranging from high to low on a continuum) in life by creating routines or rituals (i.e., also ranging on a continuum from stopping to get coffee every morning at McDonald's to celebrating a rite of passage in a specific way). In play therapy, children develop comfort routines. Comfort routines are referred to as a predictable routine(s) involving play or series of events children engage in during the session. Comfort routines are used to establish an operative level of safety in the playroom (i.e., used to create an initial safety while acclimating to the playroom and therapist, as well as maintaining an ongoing safety that is sometimes needed prior to or after engaging in certain thematic play).

Interestingly, the importance of predictability can be observed even in the midst of the unfolding of a traumatic situation, as was noticed in interviewing the children who were involved in the 1976 Chowchilla kidnapping. Terr (1990) described how many of the kidnapped children discussed that the worst moments during the kidnapping incident were during the transfer times (e.g., moving into a different vehicle, moving from the vehicle into the holding place, escaping, etc.). According to Terr, "All the transfers during the kidnapping, including the transfer from captivity to freedom, were, for the children of Chowchilla, new ventures into the unknown" (p. 37).

According to Solt and Bravo (2008), providing consistency helps children to better predict what life will be like in the following three areas: (1) experiences they will undergo, (2) the responses and actions that may be needed from them, and (3) who will be there to take care of them and keep them safe. For children, primary caregivers are typically who children look to for providing an overall sense of consistency/predictability, and therefore, security in life. Solt and Bravo (2008) discussed that caregivers engender a sense of security for children by being available and accessible, providing a daily structure/routine, and establishing a certain quality of relationship. Greenspan (2002) maintained that one quality of the caregiver-child relationship that enhanced security in children should include allowing children to express and share their feelings.

With caregivers seen as the main engender of security for children, one can only imagine how the death of a caregiver can affect the overall personal security of a child. According to Melhem, Walker, Moritz, and Brent (2008), parental death affects as many as 4 percent of all children residing in a Western country. Furthermore, the authors maintained that parental death is one of the most stressful and impactful life events that can be experienced in childhood. In ranking the order of events perceived as most distressing to children and adolescents both nationally and internationally, researchers found that one of the highest ranking events included a threat to perceived security (Yamamoto, Davis, Dylak, Whittaker, Marsh, & van der Westhuizen, 1996).

## WAR IN IRAQ: JACKSON AND THE LOSS OF HIS FATHER

In 2008, there was an estimated 148,000 U.S. troops stationed in Iraq (Pessin, 2008). R. Quillin (2008) reported that "there are almost 700,000 children in the U.S. with at least one parent deployed" (p. 1). Additionally, it is estimated that approximately 19,000 children have experienced a parent injured while in the military over the past seven years (Quillin, 2008). The confirmed death count of the military involved in the War in Iraq was 4,279 as of April 2009 (Iraq Coalition Casualty Count, 2008). In the year

2004, it was estimated that over 900 U.S. children experienced the death of a parent serving in the War in Iraq (Longley, 2004). The following case is a poignant illustration of how a child who had experienced the death of his father was able to cope in play therapy. Little did I realize how much I would learn from this child ("Soldier J") about the concept of resiliency in the wake of trauma. The heroic efforts of this brave child to cope in the midst of great loss and change in his life was unmistakable.

Jackson, a seven-year-old male, was referred to counseling after what was thought to be a one-year deployment to Iraq for his father resulted in permanent absence. Four months into his father's deployment, there was an ambush on his father's pavilion. Several of the soldiers were killed and badly injured—Jackson's father was no exception. He died a few hours after the attack—his body unable to withstand the injuries. After his father's death, Jackson began exhibiting some externalizing behaviors (i.e., aggression directed toward peers, opposition and defiance at home, etc.). Profoundly grieving, Jackson's mother eventually reached out for help as Jackson's externalizing behaviors became more unmanageable and pervasive with time.

In the intake session, Jackson's mother discussed feeling concerned over Jackson's preoccupation with the military since the death of his father. I inquired about what Jackson may have heard his dad say when he talked about going to serve in the War in Iraq. Mother chuckled as she reminisced and stated, "He probably heard his dad always complaining about having to contend with the sand—he did not like sand and especially did not like getting it in his face or shoes."

The first time I met this little boy, I was struck by his sheepish grin and cavalier way of approaching the playroom. The following depicts the beginning of our time in therapy ("J" is Jackson; "T" is therapist, Dr. Solt):

> *T*: (Welcoming Jackson to the playroom, I began my usual child-centered introduction.) Jackson, this is our special playroom and in here you can play with the toys in a lot of ways you want to.
>
> *J*: (He instantly put up his hand as if to stop me from any more talking.) You got any army men in here, Ms.?
>
> *T*: Sounds like you really like to play with the army men. . . . And there is a whole basket of army toys right over there (pointing to the shelf).
>
> *J*: Yep, army men are cool . . . my dad's one ya know? (scanning the shelf)
>
> *T*: (Reflected the large amount of pride in his eyes) You are proud your dad is a soldier. (I was honored by his willingness to share his life with me in such a short period of time.)
>
> (It was then that the sad look transformed the once exuberant face. At this point, not a lot more was said to me through verbal expression. Instead, Jackson

began working diligently to set up a war scenario in the 5′ x 5′ sandbox I had in the playroom.)

*T*: (At the end of the session) I enjoyed getting to meet you today. I am so glad you got to play in here with me. I'll see you next week, Jackson.

*J*: (Nearing the waiting room where his mother sat, Jackson looked confidently at me.) Ms., you can call me "Soldier J." That is what my dad calls me!

*T*: Soldier J it is! See you next week. (Looking over at this mother, I could see the concern on her face. Upon the intake appointment, she was very concerned that Jackson still referred to his father in present-tense—as though he was still living. She was concerned that maybe he did not fully understand or grasp that his father had been killed.)

And there it began—our work together in creating a safe place that would ultimately allow this child to express and assimilate the painful and difficult changes in his life—from his father's deployment, his father's death, and the recent move he had made with his mother.

Because relational safety lends way to vulnerable expression in therapy, my initial clinical focus with Jackson was to establish a positive therapeutic relationship. According to Ted Asay and Michael Lambert (1999), the success of therapy can be attributed to various factors, including the following: (1) client/extra-therapeutic variables (40 percent); (2) therapeutic relationship (30 percent); (3) placebo, hope, and expectancy (15 percent); and model/technique factors (15 percent). In looking at these factors contributing to the outcome variance of therapy, the therapeutic relationship is the most important factor the therapist can focus on in contributing to therapy success.

The several subsequent play sessions resulted in an intense quietness and distance from the therapist, as Jackson acclimated to the room, toys, and me (therapist). He was working to establish a sense of safety by both acclimating to the new environment, as well as developing a comfort routine—one that would span throughout most of his sessions.

His comfort routine began as soon as he entered the room, in which he would go straight to the sand. He would play with the sand for quite awhile—letting the fine grains run through his fingers, raking it and spreading it all around. Then, before involving the army toys in the sand, he would build a wall out of the big bricks—so tall he would have to stand on the chair to finish the construction. Interestingly, the wall was constructed partially between me (the therapist) and the sandbox—almost as if to divide us into two parts of the room. There was a definite distinction made by the wall, but each time the wall was made angled enough so that I could still see completely what he was doing in the sandbox without moving my chair. Even in the midst of this new environment, this child found a way to create safety through the wall and yet allowed the wall to remain off-centered insofar as allowing me to have access to his vulnerable expressions and experience while playing in the army sand.

It was easy to recognize the literal quality of his play when he began creating the war scene in the sandbox. He would slowly and deliberately place each soldier, fortress, and tank. And, when the five minute warning to end therapy was announced, he would report quietly, "No time to fight this one, maybe next time" or "No war today." Through this, I was reminded that it the often the journey and not the destination of the child's play that is significant in play therapy (Landreth, 2002). I sensed, however, from Jackson that it was inevitable that the war would occur—as soon as his security in the therapeutic relationship was established.

On the seventh session, as I walked out to greet Jackson, I was surprised to see him ("Soldier J") dressed in full uniform. Looking embarrassed, his mother explained that it was Jackson's idea to dress up in camouflage and bring his necessary gear. Smiling at Jackson, it was touching to see that he was able spend his time preparing on the outside what the inside of his heart so deeply wrestled with.

*J*: (As we entered the playroom, he ran to the puppet theater and hid behind it.) Today's a big day!

*T*: Sounds like we are in for something special!

*J*: No . . . no, *not* "special." (pause) Don't you know *anything* about war?

*T*: (Hearing his irritation and suddenly realizing he was planning to actually have a war in the playroom today—which would be anything but special to him as it claimed his father's life.) You sure seem to know a lot about war . . . maybe you could teach me some things too.

*J*: Yah, maybe . . . but could we just play in here today?

*T*: (Returning the responsibility to him) This is your time in here—you get to decide, Jackson.

*J*: No, no, no! I told you to call me *Soldier J*! (he yelled)

*T*: That was frustrating to you! Thanks for reminding me Soldier J . . . can tell that's pretty important to you! (The safety he was beginning to internalize in the therapeutic relationship was slowly allowing the scared, confused, and angry emotions to manifest—which is essential for expression and reorganization.)

He slowly walked over to the sandbox and started to prepare the war again. This time, unlike the previous sessions, the war in the sandbox actually began. It was time to use the security and safety gained from the relational predictability to enter into a new state of play that required an unparalleled amount of strength and bravery. Jackson began the war. There in the middle of bombs exploding, jeeps and tanks flipping out of the sand box due to the explosions, soldiers falling over everywhere, and some soldiers running away, Jackson grabbed his favorite soldier . . . the one he had gravitated to since the first day he saw it in the playroom. He began burying him in the sand. Clinically, I was thinking the burial of the soldier had to represent the death of his father. However, keeping him in the lead, Jackson showed me a lot more than just my mere clinical speculation:

> *J*: (Working carefully to bury the soldier deep in the sand)
>
> *T*: He's going way under there.
>
> *J*: Yah, he is trying to hide from the bad guys. He keeps getting sand in face . . . he really hates that. He really doesn't like the sand but he *has* to hide from the bad guys (continuing to cover the buried soldier with sand).
>
> *T*: He doesn't like it but he's trying hard to keep safe.
>
> *J*: Yep, he wants to go home.
>
> *T*: He knows right where he'd rather be.
>
> *J*: Yep, but they find him anyway. He doesn't know where to go now.
>
> *T*: Trying to figure out what to do next.
>
> *J*: He's is in big trouble cause the bad guys are mean and took his gun. . . . Zhoom! . . . Super shields to the rescue! Wings get ready! There he goes . . . they [the bad guys] didn't know he could fly! See ya'll later I'm going home! (The toy soldier bolted straight up into the air, away from the other toy soldiers identified as "bad guys." Jackson again found a way to fly his dad out of the middle of the sand, away from the bad guys, to where he wanted dad to be—home. Once again, he was able to grant in the fantasy of his play what could not be satisfied in the reality of his life [Landreth, 2002].)

Different scenarios like this happened for a while in therapy—dad escaping the middle of the war to come home. However, on the 13th session, he began the war and left the soldier buried. There seemed to be no need for an escape route or to act out in fantasy that the soldier was safe—it was clear that Jackson's inner strength was beginning to embrace the reality of his father's death. Consequently, his play began to overly vacillate within the typical stages of the grieving process for quite awhile as the reorganization of self continued. Over time, Jackson no longer engaged rigidly in his comfort routines and no longer constructed a wall between the therapist and the sandbox. He also began focusing less of his time playing with the army toys. He was slowly able to engage in a variety of play—generally now engaging in constructive or developmentally mastery play.

To further augment Jackson's progress, Mother was referred for filial therapy training—as she was also in a less deconstructive place with her grief and could now focus more on Jackson's needs. As Jackson continued to progress and maintain positive behavioral change outside of therapy, plans of termination were set in motion. The 19th session was the last session. In this session, Jackson brought a picture into the playroom. It contained two people (one bigger than the other), holding hands. He had drawn the letter "I," a heart, and the letter "U" between the two people (i.e., saying, "I Love You"). After he showed me his picture, he instantly went to the sandbox and buried it carefully under the sand. "You knew exactly where you wanted that picture to be," I responded. Grinning, he turned to me and said, "Ms. Misty, can we work on building a bridge?" For the remainder of the last session, we created a variety of bridges out of the numerous cardboard bricks in the playroom. Consistent with and representative of his world—he had created a bridge from one side of grief to the other. Although the memory of his father lived on—the war had subsided.

## 9/11: DARIA AND THE LOSS OF HER MOTHER

If predictability leads to a feeling of safety, it is no wonder how terrifyingly unsafe the nation felt during and after the terrorist attacks against our country on September 11, 2001. According to Karen Seeley (2008), "terrorists attacks, which are deliberately designed to provoke intense fear, shock, and intimidation among the population at large, are perhaps the most psychologically harmful of all disasters" (p. 11). Approximately 2,749 people were killed in the 9/11 terrorist attacks in New York (Seeley, 2008). It was further estimated that 3,051 children experienced the death of a parent in the 9/11 attacks (New York Media, 2009).

Providing enough mental health resources needed to address such monumental loss seemed to be a Herculean endeavor. By the end of the fourth week following 9/11, the American Red Cross had made over 61,104 mental health contacts (American Red Cross, 2001). Seeley (2008) reported that the cases of depression and posttraumatic stress disorder almost doubled in Manhattan after the 9/11 attacks. Terence Gorski (2001) estimated that the ratio of grievers per deceased in the 9/11 attack was 18 to 1. Additionally, Gorski maintained that 5 out of these 18 individuals would experience complicated, prolonged grief (i.e., often involving posttraumatic stress disorder), which would require outside assistance such as counseling.

In Texas, I joined a team of other area child therapists and traveled to New York to offer assistance to the children who experienced parental death as a result of the 9/11 attacks. Having had years of training and supervision in both crisis counseling and trauma, I was ready to begin my work. It didn't take long for me to realize just how much more I would learn about survival and resilience from the children and families who lost so much in such a short time.

We were stationed in the crisis shelter established at Pier 94, named the Family Assistance Center. Walking into the Family Assistance Center and looking at what seemed to be a three-mile-long memorial wall of pictures and updates on missing or deceased loved ones, the magnitude of loss was overwhelming. Little did I know I would be visiting that memorial wall with almost every child I worked with in the Family Assistance Center. To the children, that memorial wall was the predictable, concrete place in which their mother/father remained—not to mention it was the representation of hope should any news of their loved one materialize. It was the gathering spot for many and was the ultimate encapsulation of the strength and resiliency of the individuals who experienced the death of a loved one due to 9/11.

Stationed toward the back in the Family Assistance Center was the designated children's area where caregivers were able to leave children for certain lengths of time to take care of necessary business (i.e., rendering DNA testing, filing for unemployment, locating shelter, etc.). This could also be a time for a (now) single caregiver to grieve and talk to a trained mental health professional by him- or herself. That being said, it understandably was hours before some of the children were retrieved.

Trained mental health professionals helped staff the designated children's area. This area contained a plethora of activities and crafts for the children to engage should they desire. There were also a lot of toys entailing the following general toy categories used in play therapy: creative expressive, dramatic, real-life, nurturing, aggressive, and general developmental mastery. The time spent with each child varied significantly (i.e., some children were seen daily over the span of a week and some children only once; some children staying for hours and some for only 15 minutes). The following is a story that illustrates the heroism of one child in the wake of trauma.

Daria had just turned six years of age weeks before the 9/11 attack. Her mother worked in the North Twin Tower. Shortly after her grandmother checked her into the children's area, she quickly found a corner and hid under the several of the stuffed animals. I eagerly volunteered to be assigned to Daria during her undetermined length of stay. Although she appeared quiet and frightened, she had a presence of strength about her that was unmistakable.

As she managed to hide her entire lower body, I tracked her diligent effort, by saying ("D" is Daria; "T" is Therapist, Dr. Solt):

*T*: You are working really hard to hide under all of those (stuffed animals).

(She was working meticulously to hide every small area of herself.)

*T*: Covering up each part of yourself.

As time went on and no more animals where in her reach, she had the confidence to ask for some help from me and in a barely audible voice:

*D*: Can you hand me more animals please?

*T*: You're still working hard and want me to help so the other animals don't fall off (handing the animals to her one-by-one).

*D*: (She nodded and continued to work) Will you cover up my head with these? (pointing to the animals left on the floor)

*T*: You want to be completely covered. You don't want anyone to see you (as I carefully placed the animals around the top of her head).

(She stayed quiet for about a minute.)

*T*: It feels good to be hidden. You seem to like staying in here.

*D*: (Still quiet, not making a sound.)

*T*: You made a place where you feel safe (thinking, of course that she was creating a sense of safety in light of all she had been through and to escape the novelty of the children's area. After another minute, I heard her giggle and start to move.).

*T*: I hear you moving under there.

(Then, I saw her left hand and arm reach up through the animals.)

*D*: I am here, right here!

*T*: You wanted to let me know exactly where you are.

*D*: Yes, I am right here! You found me! I was way under there!

*T*: You're excited you were found! It feels good to be found and know you are safe.

(Realizing now that what she was playing out was exactly what her grandmother had reported to an attendant when she checked Daria into the children's area. Grandmother had discussed still holding onto hope that Daria's mother would eventually be found in the rubble so that they could "put her body to rest." She then popped out of all the animals and moved over to the building blocks. Carefully one by one she stacked the blocks until she had constructed a tall building.)

*D*: Do you know what happens if it gets too tall?

*T*: Umm, sounds like you might know.

*D*: It falls over everywhere and people can get stuck and stuck (has a very sad look on her face).

*T*: Feels really sad to think about that.

*D*: Yeah, cause that is where my mama is, she is stuck real good under the buildin'. She can't get out 'cause the buildin' is real big (displaying a really sad look with tears in her eyes—her hurt was unmistakable).

*T*: You really miss your mom . . . you feel so sad right now thinking about her and all that's happened.

(And, then the rescue began. She began working diligently to remove each block and put them in a pile.)

*D*: We're almost there . . . almost to the bottom (as she worked hard to reach the bottom).

*T*: You are working hard to clear each block away.

*D*: (Reaching the end of the pile, she turned and looked at me) I can show what my mama looks like if you want to see. (This was the first trip to the memorial wall with Daria—and many more were to come during the week she came to the children's area.)

Daria's inner strength and bravery to instantaneously express her fears and loss through her play was admirable. Plato once said, "You can discover more about a person in an hour of play than in a year of conversation." And although I had just met Daria, through her play, she was willing and able to show me the pain and hardship of her perception of the recent tragedy involving her mother. There was no grandiose technique to employ to make Daria's life different than what it was in this moment (i.e., to rid her of the pain or to bring her mother back). Her ability to embrace the reality of this pain and share this with someone was a testament to her presence of strength.

The clinical focus I maintained during my brief time with Daria involved employing a child-centered approach (i.e., expressing warmth, empathy, and understanding through reflection and tracking skills). Badenoch (2008) discussed how responses of this nature can engender a sense of being seen and heard, which ultimately results in facilitating the formation of connections between the middle prefrontal and limbic areas in the brain. Badenoch further reported that when children are able to express various feelings and needs with their therapist, integration between the child's right and left brain hemispheres occurs, assisting in the overall calming of the limbic circuits.

Over the course of the week, Daria disclosed and revealed some painful thoughts, fears, and questions she had regarding what mom may have endured in her last moments. Her strength to stand by her mother's picture that hung on the memorial wall and reminisce about her birthday party that mom planned just weeks before was profound. Daria's ability to build up and hold her mother's memory was much more powerful than the force of the falling Twin Tower that brought her mom to her death.

## HURRICANE KATRINA: GARRETT AND THE LOSS OF HIS HOME

Hurricane Katrina, which occurred in August of 2005, was deemed the costliest and third deadliest storm in the history of the United States (Weather Channel, 2007). Approximately 1.2 million people were under an evacuation order and the total amount of deaths that resulted from Hurricane Katrina (both direct and indirect) was 1,833 (Weather Channel, 2007). While local residents had prepared for numerous hurricanes before—only for them to be less intense than anticipated—Hurricane Katrina lived true to its prognostication and shocked the nation with its devastation.

Working on the crisis team for our local school district, I became involved in the effort to help the child Hurricane Katrina evacuees that had entered our school district. My job was to provide brief crisis counseling to the children for stabilization purposes. While there were varying coping styles observed from the children, they all seemed to still be in a state of disbelief over the events that had so suddenly occurred. Diana Sullivan Everstine and Louis Everstine (1993) described an individual's lack of preparedness as the main forerunner to a trauma response, and therefore, yielding disbelief as one of the most immediate feelings to take place in the emotional sequelae following a traumatic event. Consequently, the initial assistance in helping the children and families affected by Hurricane Katrina was letting them process their disbelief over the storm, resulting in the massive amount of devastation that it caused. The following story is one example of the many children that coped with a significant amount of loss and change in the aftermath of Katrina.

Garrett, a seven-year-old male, had been displaced from his home in New Orleans due to Hurricane Katrina. Having been a native to New Orleans, contending with hurricanes was part of life for Garrett and his family. Once his family decided to evacuate, there was very little time to pack anything of importance. Garrett was instructed to pack a set of clothes, pajamas, his piggy bank, and a few toys in his backpack. That was all—no time to grab anything else as time was of the essence in regard to safety.

The first few weeks in his (suddenly) new home and school, Garrett did relatively okay—as he seemed to be adjusting to the disruption that occurred in his life. He was struggling to stay focused on schoolwork and appeared uninterested in socializing with peers, but otherwise pleasant and compliant at home and in the classroom. Upon the fourth week of his new school, however, a peer mistakenly took Garrett's backpack, which resulted in a less than ideal reaction from Garrett. After assaulting his classmate in the process of retrieving his backpack, he collapsed on top of the backpack into a fetal-like position, sobbing uncontrollably. After several minutes turned into an hour of crying, it was clear that this little boy—willing to protect at all costs what little possessions he had left—was profoundly grieving the catastrophe he recently experienced in his life.

I started seeing Garrett twice a week in individual play therapy during the first month of therapy. The first several sessions with Garrett involved a lot of aggressive play. The anger he displayed was infused in most all interactions with me and the toys. Several times within the session, Garrett would take the play sword and stab at the dollhouse, knocking furniture over and even out of the house. Eventually, before he left, the dollhouse would be empty and all the furniture would be strewn throughout the playroom floor. With this much aggression and intensity occurring each week in the playroom, interestingly, at school he was back to the status quo of behaving in a pleasant, compliant manner. On the sixth session, after knocking all the furniture out of the house, Garrett found the little suitcase in the playroom over by the dress-up clothes. (G=Garrett; T: Therapist, Dr. Solt)

> *G*: (In a matter-of-fact way) It's time to pack.
>
> *T*: You're getting ready for something.
>
> *G*: Yeah. You need to pack too.
>
> *T*: Sounds like we may be going somewhere.
>
> *G*: Maybe, but I'm not sure where. You just better hurry. And don't forget the cat! (He was quickly shoving some dress-up clothes, play food, and some money from the cash register into his suitcase. Then, he grabbed the large stuffed cat and shoved it also into the suitcase.)

About the time he finished packing, it was time for the session to end. His theme had progressed from empting the house, making a mess of the contents all around the room, to now packing a suitcase with necessities. Trying to enter into his phenomenological view, I deeply pondered what I knew about what happened that day for him and his family. According to Everstine and Everstine (1993), in assisting a person in their recovery from trauma, the therapist must consider that trauma is both event-specific and that it is driven by the person's "personal significance of that event" (p. 13). Garrett was bravely showing me his perspective of exactly what had happened and what had changed his life so significantly—that his home and most all of his belongings, which represented a sense of permanency and constancy, had been literally washed away by the tumultuous rain and flooding inflicted by Hurricane Katrina.

Unfortunately, around the time of that session, Texas began experiencing inclement weather for several consecutive weeks (i.e., thunderstorms, wind, tornado warnings, and periods of heavy flooding due to the continuous rains). Garrett, like many of the children I was working with in therapy who had survived Hurricane Katrina, began experiencing heightened symptoms of anxiety. The similar sensory experiences related to the inclement weather in Texas triggered immediate associations to the unfolding of Hurricane Katrina. To better stabilize Garrett during this time, I began meeting with Garrett's mother in separate parent consultations one time per week. While we discussed interventions to employ at home in hopes of increased feelings of safety for Garrett during the inclement weather, I began to learn more about just how tragic the moments were for the family during their escape from New Orleans to Texas.

While being in denial initially, his mother began opening up to me with what was described as "The worst day of my life—which is now a prolonged reality." Natives to New Orleans, the hurricane was not perceived as an imminent threat to the family, as they had several warnings through the years which turned out to be nonproductive. Therefore, when the advisory to leave was announced, it was taken lightly for quite some time. When they finally decided to leave, the parents quickly packed and were out of the house within 30 minutes. As they were pulling away, a large tree was blown onto their home. As they drove away, another small tree fell onto their car. As they neared the end of their road, mother reported that Garrett started to cry over having to leave the cat (a transient neighborhood cat that he played with frequently). With the amount of devastation and loss swirling around them, they took a plight into the unknown and ended in Frisco, Texas. It was no doubt a life-altering day for the entire family.

As the weather became calmer again in Texas, so did Garrett's anxiety. Interestingly, during the inclement weather, he manifested different play from before—in that he neither displayed aggression nor targeted the dollhouse or suitcase—he just played quietly and very constrictively. Once the storms seemed to subside, he once again began ridding the dollhouse of its furniture and packing the suitcase with supplies. Upon session 12, however, he quickly packed his basic supplies, closed up the suitcase, and hid it under the bean bag.

> G: Don't move this anywhere, and if anybody else finds it tell them to leave it alone (stating this is a demanding voice).
>
> *T*: You found a place to keep your things safe and it's important to know they'll be there when you come back.
>
> G: Yah, so don't let any other kid come and take it.
>
> *T*: (Knowing the impossibility of leaving the items there due to seeing several more children in a week's time) Garrett, I know you want them to be left right there, but other boys and girls play with the toys too. All the toys will be in their spots for you when you come in again so you can find them.
>
> G: Okay, I guess I will get them next time if I have to.

It is important, especially when working with traumatized children, that the child counseling office/playroom is kept as predictable as possible. This room becomes the emotional container of predictability by which a sense of safety is engendered. This predictability includes ensuring the toys are returned to the exact same location, including even small items, such as the dollhouse furniture (Landreth, 2002). It is also important to communicate expectations and limits to children in regard to the therapy room. While it would have been easy for me to acquiesce to Garrett's request of leaving the suitcase, it would have been a bigger disappointment and frustration for him to check and it not be there next week. That would have diminished his safety in the therapeutic relationship which is the foundation by which the therapy takes place. The playroom does provide anchors to reality—and the fact that other children use the room is a reality.

My work with Garrett continued for 17 sessions. At the end of therapy, it was clear that he was ready to terminate as he was showing signs of adjustment (i.e., demonstrating greater ego strength and self-concept, improving grades, and reciprocating socially). In therapy, Garrett's play had indicated several emotional shifts. He had begun to engage in constructive play within the dollhouse—arranging the furniture in the rooms instead of wreaking havoc. He also ceased the packing of the suitcase play. Upon the 14th session, after he packed his suitcase and hid it under the bean bag, he returned to it at the end of the session. One by one, he placed the items back on the shelves (but not in their original locations) as he talked about a birthday party he was invited to by one of his classmates. Metaphorically, that did represent his life: he packed, he hid (internally), and he unpacked his life in a new location with a new home, friends, and environment. In spite of the devastation Hurricane Katrina inflicted upon this young boy, his strength and courage brought him to dry land.

## CONCLUSION

The incredible strength, courage, and determination I have observed in working with countless children coping with trauma and loss over the past 12 years is both humbling and encouraging. The bravery of these children and families to face such life-altering adversity in hopes of discovering a new paradigm necessary for continued existence is beyond words. How courageous and heroic they are.

## REFERENCES

American Red Cross (2001). American Red Cross in greater New York. Retrieved March 11, 2009, from http://www.nyredcross.org/media/ar2001_timeline.pdf.

Asay, T. P., & Lambert, M. J. (1999). The empirical case for the common factors in therapy: Quantitative findings. In M. A. Hubble, B. L. Duncan, & S. D. Miller (Eds.), *The heart and soul of change: What works in therapy* (pp. 33–56). Washington, DC: American Psychological Association.

Badenoch, B. (2008). *Being a brain-wise therapist: A practical guide to interpersonal neurobiology*. New York: W. W. Norton & Company.

Crenshaw, D. A. (2008). *Therapeutic engagement of children and adolescents: Play, symbol, drawing, and storytelling strategies*. New York: Jason Aronson.

Everstine, D. S., & Everstine, L. (1993). *The trauma response: Treatment for emotional injury*. New York: W. W. Norton & Company.

Gorski, T. T. (2001). Incidence of PTSD after terrorist attacks. Retrieved January 18, 2009, from http://www.tgorski.com/terrorism/PTSD_Incidence_After_Terrorist_Attacks.htm.

Greenspan, S. I. (2002). *The secure child: Helping children feel safe and confident in a changing world*. Cambridge, MA: Persus Publishing.

Iraq Coalition Casualty Count (2008). iCasualties.org. Retrieved on March 13, 2009, from http://icasualties.org/Iraq/index/aspx.

Landreth, G. L. (2002). *Play therapy: The art of the relationship*. New York: Brunner-Routledge.

Longley, J. (Producer & Director), & Sinno, J. (Producer). (2004). *Iraq in fragments* [Documentary film]. United States: Typecast Pictures.

Melhem, N. M., Walker, M., Moritz, G., & Brent, D. A. (2008). Antecedent and sequelae of sudden parental death in offspring and surviving caregivers. *Archives of Pediatrics and Adolescent Medicine, 162*(5), 403–410. Retrieved March 15, 2009, from http://archpedi.ama- assn.org/cgi/content/full/162/5/403.

New York Media (2009). 9/11 by the numbers. Retrieved on February 3, 2009, from http://nymag.com/nymetro/new/sept11/features/n_7692/.

Pessin, A. (2008). As Surge ends, how many U.S. troops will remain in Iraq. *Voice of America*. Retrieved March 8, 2009, from http://www.voanews.com/english/archive/2008-07.

Quillin, R. (2008). Camp C.O.P.E. helps military kids deal with effects of war. Retrieved on January 7, 2009, from http://www.eclubamerica.com/index.php?option=com_content&task.

Seeley, K. M. (2008). *Therapy after terror: 9/11, psychotherapists, and mental health*. New York: Cambridge University Press.

Solt, M., & Bravo, S. (2008, Fall). Children adjusting to a caregiver's military deployment. *Association for Play Therapy Newsletter, 3*, 16–18.

Terr, L. (1990). *Too scared to cry: How trauma affects children . . . and ultimately us all*. New York: Basic Books.

Terr, L. (1994). *Unchained memories: True stories of traumatic memories, lost and found*. New York: Basic Books.

The Weather Channel (2007). Katrina's statistics tell story of its wrath. Retrieved March 11, 2009, from http://www.weather.com/newscenter/topstories/060829katrinastats.html.

Yamamoto, K., Davis, O., Dylak, S., Whittaker, J., Marsh, C., & van der Westhuizen, P. C. (1996). Across six nations: Stressful events in the lives of children. *Child Psychiatry and Human Development, 26*(3), 139–149.

# III

# STRENGTHS-BASED APPLICATIONS IN ASSESSMENT, TRAINING, AND TREATMENT COLLABORATION

# 13

# A Strengths-Based Approach to Assessment

*Lenore Strocchia-Rivera*

The task of identifying strengths is relatively easy to do when conducting psychological assessments, for as the psychologist inquires about so many different facets of a person's life, strengths and talents peek out in all kinds of places and at different points in time throughout the person's life. Even when a person has faced a lifetime of trauma and hardship, there are often factors at work that have held that person up. One of these is usually an adult who provided unwavering support to the person in need. The fact that the person in need was able to endear himself or herself to this supportive adult is without doubt a strength in itself. The question before the assessor, then, is how will these identified strengths be honored? What place and how much importance will they be given in the feedback session? In the report?

The challenge of providing a strengths-based assessment is being able to provide a balanced and comprehensive portrait of the person in order to answer questions posed by (1) the assessed and (2) the referral source, if the assessed did not self-refer. Developing a balanced portrait has always been more difficult for me to do when conducting an evaluation, rather than an assessment, for the referral source (e.g., school, court, company) typically wants to know more about the deficit areas of functioning in order to determine eligibility of the person for a particular outcome (e.g., special education program, services, jobs, legal dispositions) than the areas of strength. Assessments, on the other hand, are typically concerned with strengthening or enhancing the goodness of fit between the individual and the tasks they are encountering in their current role or setting. Suitability, rather than eligibility, for certain services and jobs is the general aim.

According to Stephen Finn (2007), traditional (or information-gathering) assessments are different from therapeutic assessments, where the former involves an "expert" assessor carefully collecting standardized test data in order to diagnose, plan or evaluate treatment, and/or increase understanding. The latter is what Finn (2007) calls an "attitude about psychological assessment" where the goal is to create a positive experience and to help create positive changes in patients and in those individuals who have a stake in their lives (such as parents and therapists). This type of assessment intends to help patients *directly* rather than indirectly, as with traditional assessment.

Finn (2007) further breaks down "therapeutic assessments" into those that can be considered collaborative or noncollaborative. For instance, Finn cites Paul Lerner (2005) as an example of a gifted psychologist who positively impacted clients through assessments without ever explicitly asserting that they were therapeutic. On the other hand, collaborative assessments are "a comprehensive effort to engage the client in multiple phases of the assessment process, including (a) framing the reasons for the assessment, (b) observing test responses and behaviors, (c) discovering the significance of those responses and behaviors, (d) coming up with useful recommendations, and (e) drafting summary documents at the end" (p. 5). Three pioneers of this method are Fischer (1985/1994), Handler (2007), and Purves (2002), and each tried to make the assessment process more humane, respectful, and understandable to clients (Finn, 2007).

One type of collaborative assessment is called Therapeutic Assessment (upper case), originated and popularized by Steve Finn of the Center for Therapeutic Assessment in Austin, Texas. Therapeutic Assessment is a semi-structured form of collaborative assessment that is actually a clinical (i.e., brief therapy) method whose explicit goal is to leave clients positively changed at the end of the assessment (Tharinger et al., 2007). Throughout this chapter, I will differentiate between a generic strengths-based mind-set when conducting assessments and more specific types of therapeutic assessments whenever necessary.

## ADVANTAGES OF A STRENGTHS-BASED MIND-SET IN CONDUCTING ASSESSMENTS

The advantages of a strengths-based mind-set in conducting assessments are multifold. For one, it allows clients to feel empowered with making changes. The mother of a former child client once wrote me and said that the strengths-based approach I used "conveyed a sense of accessible power and acceptance." I immediately liked the term "accessible power" because the ultimate goal of a therapeutic assessment is to meet the individual goals and/or needs of the client, and what better way to do that than to help clients feel empowered to make whatever changes are necessary to achieve their end goal or satisfy their needs.

Another advantage of a strengths-based mind-set when conducting assessments is that the assessor is more likely to obtain valid data. A study by Finn and Tonsager (1992) found that when clients were treated as collaborators in the assessment process, and time was taken to solicit what *they* wanted to learn about themselves from the assessment, test results came back as more valid (i.e., profiles were deemed "less defensive") than when they were not treated as collaborators.

## ADVANTAGES OF THERAPEUTIC ASSESSMENT

As stated in Deborah Tharinger et al. (2007) a particular advantage of Therapeutic Assessment is that it produces positive treatment effects (Finn & Tonsager, 1992; Newman & Greenway, 1997). Among college student subjects, these included decreased symptomatology, greater self-esteem, and increased hopefulness. Also as cited in Tharinger et al. (2007), another study by Ackerman, Hilsenroth, Baity, and Blagys (2000) found that after Therapeutic Assessment, adult clients were more likely to complete recommended treatment and feel a stronger alliance with their assessor than clients who received a traditional psychological assessment. Moreover, Hilsenroth, Peters, and Ackerman (2004), as also cited in Tharinger et al. (2007), replicated this finding and showed that the positive benefits extended to the alliance clients developed with their therapists in subsequent treatment.

Therapeutic Assessment can also result in enhanced parental efficacy (Tharinger, Finn, & Austin et al., 2008) and, in my experience, higher levels of patience from parents toward children. For example, many parents refer their children for an assessment because of oppositional behavior. When the results of an assessment indicate attention-deficit hyperactivity disorder (ADHD) and suggest that the child has difficulty following through on directives because of a brief auditory attention span and/or deficient working memory, the result is usually one of increased compassion and hopefulness due to the availability of effective ADHD treatments. Similarly, if a child has been referred for an assessment due to suspected ADHD but there is insufficient evidence to support this kind of diagnosis, the assessor may be able to point to alternative explanations for the child's behavior. As discussed in Finn (2003) and consistent with my experience, anxiety related to trauma produces many of the same symptoms associated with ADHD; if the assessment produces elevated scores on trauma-related behavior scales, then introducing the idea of trauma-based behaviors as a possible explanation for the ADHD-like symptoms often leads to a helpful (and sometimes first) dialogue between parent and child around the traumatic incident(s).

## QUALITY ASSESSMENTS AS FUNDAMENTAL

Though it may seem obvious, in order for any assessment or evaluation to be helpful in guiding treatment interventions or serve as a therapeutic intervention, it must rest upon a well-done assessment. I would like to briefly touch upon the elements of a quality assessment before discussing further how a Therapeutic Assessment can produce desired change in a client. These include accurately executing the assessment, deeply listening to clients, and tailoring recommendations to clients and those who have a stake in their lives.

### A Good Foundation

The ability of the assessor to accurately administer, score, and interpret the tests used during the assessment provides the foundation for a quality assessment. An incorrectly administered, erroneously scored, or wrongly interpreted test will obviously undermine any of the findings and recommendations of the assessor while, conversely, one that is executed well on these basic levels will serve as a good foundation. In my 20 years of supervising psychological evaluations and assessments, I have found that an assessor's professional degree or years of experience in the field has little to do with the quality of administration, scoring, and interpretation. Instead, the factors that appear to explain most of the variance in this area are: (a) the amount of training and experience an assessor has had with a particular test; (b) the assessor's tendency to be careful and mindful of all standardized procedures; and (c) the assessor's willingness (and humbleness) to double-check one's administration, scoring, and/or interpretation whenever there is a hint of something in the assessment not looking right.

As will be expounded upon later in this chapter, it is critically important to engage the client and his or her parents in the interpretation process. Is a particular assessment finding an anomaly in the face of previous findings? How well does the finding fit with what they know to be true about the individual? If there is a discrepancy in findings from the current and previous assessments, how can this discrepancy be reconciled? Certainly there will be times when it cannot be, but it is incumbent upon the assessor to acknowledge the discrepancy and address it to the best of his or her ability.

### Effective Listening

The ability of the assessor to listen carefully and deeply to the concerns of the client (and his or her parents) so that the referral questions are clear and understood by all involved parties is another factor related to high-quality assessment work. Germane to this, the assessor is wise to take a collaborative approach, designing the assessment process around the questions that are most prominently on the minds of the assessed (and his or her parents).

### Empathy

This refers to the ability of the assessor to empathize with the pain and suffering of the individual (and his or her parents who may suffer along with them) seeking the assessment. Finn (2007) believes that a good assessment can serve as an "empathy magnifier" for the assessor.

### Tailored Recommendations

Meaningful and doable recommendations are perhaps the most crucial part of the assessment process. If such recommendations are not tailored to the needs of the clients and the important caretakers in their lives, the assessment process can be construed not just as frustrating, but as a sign of disrespect for the time and money of those who entrusted them to the assessor. Thus, the creation of meaningful and doable recommendations depends in part on the knowledge base of the assessor so that he or she can draw upon current research findings, especially those related to evidence-based treatment approaches.

Below are some ideas on how to make results and recommendations meaningful to different audiences. Communicating these recommendations with respect to the audience's needs, goals, and developmental capacities is likely to facilitate rather than frustrate their implementation. In all cases, however, I attempt to provide both oral and written feedback, as research by Lance and Krishnamurthy (2003), as cited by Finn (2007), demonstrated that a combination of oral and written feedback was superior to oral feedback alone.

## CHILDREN

For children, an oral (followed by written) explanation of results via a metaphorical story appears to be the most effective and helpful way to convey answers to the questions they have generated with the help of their parents and the assessor. When the story is presented in written form, the child has an opportunity to read and reread answers to their assessment questions and it can serve as a long-term support to their ego development. The beautiful thing about a written story is that the author can project into the future questions that the child may ask about his difficulties, and the story can offer reaffirming responses in anticipation of those questions.

When presented as a hardcover book, as can be done through the children's activity kit *Illustory* (commercially available through Chimeric, Inc.), the child is usually excited to read a story that portrays him or her as the main character!

Alternatively, depending on the developmental capacity of the child, the child and assessor can co-create the metaphorical story during play therapy sessions. At the end of therapy, the child can be presented with a written account of the story. Whether created solely by the assessor, the child, parents, or some combination of these individuals, such a creation can be treasured for years to come. For examples of how a therapeutic story (or fables) can be used to share results with children, see Tharinger, Finn, Wilkinson, and DeHay et al. (2008).

## ADOLESCENTS

For adolescents, I like to use letters crafted in the spirit and tradition of the late, renowned psychotherapist Michael White (cf. White & Epston, 1990). White's belief is that long after a report has been written up, it's the letters that get read and reread by the people whose lives are directly touched by the evaluation or assessment. In his letters, he takes the time to reiterate his validation of the person's struggles, their strengths, and reasons for hopefulness. In my letters, I attempt to include these elements along with a more elaborate explanation of *why*, based on the assessment findings unique to that person, what he or she seems to be struggling with, and what he or she might consider doing differently in the future to guard against continuing frustrations and disappointments. The written word usually proves to be quite powerful.

However, the empathic tone of the written word is probably what accounts for the letter's enduring power. I always strive to use a tone and convey an attitude that would honor Michael White, and here I would like to add a word or two about Michael and his philosophy of healing as beautifully recounted by his longtime colleague, David Epston.

In one of his posted speeches, entitled *Remembering Michael White*, David wrote that Michael was strongly influenced by the philosopher Michel Foucault. In a book chapter about Foucault, philosopher Philip Caputo wrote that although Foucault was not a therapist, if he did invent a therapy, it would *not* look

> at the mad as patients in the sense of objects of medical knowledge but as "patiens," as ones who suffer greatly, who suffer from their knowledge. Such a patient would not be an object of knowledge but an author or subject of knowledge, one from whom we have something to learn. (cited in Epston, 2008, p. 4)

Caputo went on to surmise that for Foucault as a therapist,

> The healing gesture meant to heal this suffering is not intended to explain it away or fill in the abyss but simply to affirm that they are not alone, that our common madness is a matter of degree, that we're all siblings in the same night of truth. The healing gesture is not to explain madness if that means to explain it away but to recognize it as a common fate, to affirm our community and solidarity. (cited in Epston, 2008, p. 4)

David compares this to his abstract of a quote from Michael in 1993:

> And what of solidarity? I am thinking of a solidarity that is constructed by therapists who refuse to draw a sharp distinction between their lives and the lives of others, who refuse to marginalize those persons who seek help, by therapists who are constantly confronting the fact that if faced with the circumstances such that provide the context of troubles of others, they just might not be doing nearly as well themselves. (cited in Epston, 2008, p. 5)

Thus, the tone of my letter attempts to convey my fundamental belief that if I were in my client's shoes, I may not be doing any better than she is doing right now.

## PARENTS

As with teens, letters can be given to parents so that they answer questions posed for the assessment. Other parents prefer to get the whole report if the questions they posed are the same ones posed by another referral source, such as a school. For both parents and teens, including contact information for recommended treatment providers and the names of different treatment approaches greatly facilitates follow-through. It also helps when my letter or report gets passed on to the next treatment provider so that the rationale for my recommendations is clearly understood.

## FAMILIES

Sharing tentative results of a child assessment during a family session provides the assessor with an opportunity to "observe the child in a family context, test systemic hypotheses, better understand the meaning of individual test results, and try out possible interventions" (Tharinger, Finn, & Austin et al., 2008, p. 547). Tharinger, Finn, and Austin et al. (2008) found through years of research that a family session may help parents see systemic aspects of their child's problems, help the child feel less blamed, foster positive experiences among family members, and offer the family a glimpse of family therapy. Such a family session can be fraught with anxiety and stress as parents are prone to blaming themselves for their children's behavior difficulties. For this reason, it is critical that assessors think carefully about how to communicate findings so that they are helpful and not harmful. Tharinger, Finn, and Austin et al. (2008) wrote an excellent article about how to consider the various factors that inevitably impinge on a successful family session.

The specific technique an assessor may choose to use for communicating findings, of course, should depend on what the assessor is trying to accomplish in service of the clients' needs and goals. An assessor who is proficient in the many family therapy methods and techniques is best equipped to handle such a session. Several approaches, such as family drawing, semi-structured play, parent coaching/skill development, psychodrama, Consensus TAT, Consensus Rorschach, and family sculpture, are outlined in Tharinger, Finn, and Hersh et al. (2008). My personal favorite is family sculpture, sometimes referred to as family reconstruction, which is an active therapy technique developed by family therapy pioneer Virginia Satir. As the term "family sculpture" suggests, family members are actively positioned by therapists to nonverbally convey dynamics in the family system, thus allowing family members to reconsider their thinking about the causes and effects of an individual's behavior and emotional difficulties.

## TEACHERS AND SCHOOLS

If the reason for referral is primarily psychoeducational in nature and special education services seem appropriate, I write a report for the school district so that Committees on Special Education (CSEs) can take results into consideration when determining eligibility for special education services. Knowing federal and state education laws helps me choose effective language in describing my results and recommendations. If special education services are not indicated or parents do not wish to pursue them, I have offered to write a one-to-two page summary letter of findings for the child's teachers.

In these cases, the tone of the letter is just as important as content. For content, I usually address the historical nature of a student's struggles by citing grades and teachers' comments from report cards as far back as kindergarten (or preschool if I can get my hands on the teacher's narratives!) and standardized test results. To me, this comprehensive and historical review conveys respect to the child's teachers who took the time to write informed comments about this child's performance in various arenas. I find that this historical overview lends an attitude of support and empathy toward both the child and the present teacher. Moreover, the focus of my recommendations is on what the student needs in order to learn optimally and to be evaluated fairly. They are neither demands nor dictates. They are, rather, offered in the spirit of trying to honor what has and has not worked well in the past. They are my way of sharing thoughts with other professionals, who have known this child for longer than I, and helping them appreciate the child's difficulties so that they can readily access their innate compassion when working with this child. Just as the assessor uses tests as "empathy magnifiers" (Finn, 2007), so does the assessor use the results and recommendations as "empathy magnifiers" for teachers.

## REFERRAL SOURCES

For referral sources, I have found that a phone or in-person follow-up is helpful. Oftentimes, the referral source has been right on the money with his hunches and is grateful for the external validation. Other times, she may have been stumped with trying to help an individual and is grateful to hear a different perspective on the problem so that she can develop new treatment angles. In both cases, it is incumbent upon me, the assessor, to realize that I had the easy job in all of this. It is the ongoing treatment provider who has the tough job of helping his or her clients reach their goals. My role is simply to offer the referral source (e.g., therapist) a new or enhanced understanding of the cumulative and/or synergistic forces standing between a client and his or her goals.

## SHOWING REVERENCE THROUGH THE THERAPEUTIC ASSESSMENT APPROACH

What sets apart Therapeutic Assessment (upper case) from therapeutic assessment (lower case), according to Finn (2007), is the semistructured nature of the assessment. Most importantly, he wrote, Therapeutic Assessment findings are initially sorted according to levels of congruency with a client's self-understanding and then presented in a specific order so that clients are most able to integrate and make use of assessment information. Finn recommends starting an assessment feedback session with Level 1 findings, followed by Level 2 findings, and finally by Level 3 findings.

Level 1 findings are those that verify clients' usual ways of thinking about themselves and that will be accepted easily in the feedback session. Finn refers to the sharing of this information as part of the "mirror process," whereby the assessor mirrors back to clients the pain and suffering they have been through. Finn (March 2009, personal communication) firmly believes that, for most clients, it is only after they have been "heard" can they hear about their strengths. For a minority of clients, the assessor can begin to share results that focus on clients' resiliency and strengths if their main self-conceptualization is focused on strengths and resiliency. If it is not, the assessor risks having an empathic break with the clients (and ultimately, those who have a stake in the client's life).

According to Finn (2007), Level 2 findings are those that modify or amplify clients' usual ways of thinking about themselves, but that are unlikely to threaten self-esteem or cherished self-perceptions. For example, Finn (2007) might tell a client who is concerned about lethargy, lack of motivation, and poor focus that his Rorschach D score of –4 suggests that he is emotionally overwhelmed, rather than just "lazy" as he fears.

Finn (2007) describes Level 3 findings as those that are so novel or discrepant from clients' usual ways of thinking about themselves that they are likely to be rejected in feedback sessions. These findings tend to provoke so much anxiety that clients are likely to employ their dominant defense mechanisms shortly after hearing them. However, as predicted by self-verification theory (e.g., Swann, 1996) and schema theory, research has shown that in many instances, clients continue to consider and assimilate such information long after an assessment is completed. By starting with Level 1 findings and gradually offering Level 2 and then Level 3 findings, assessors can help clients incorporate new information into their preexisting schemas and, if necessary, develop new schemas about themselves and their way of relating to the world.

Finn (March 2009, personal communication) has astutely pointed out that sometimes it is too difficult to know beforehand what would be considered an affirmation of a client's self-conceptualization and what would not. To guard against making a wrong guess, Finn will often begin a feedback session with the question, "What is the worst possible thing I can tell you about you (your son, your daughter)?" Once the assessor hears the client's response, he or she is better equipped to determine what result(s) are affirming to the client's self-conceptualization and, therefore, can proceed with sharing the Level 1 findings. If the assessor is wrong (e.g., giving Level 1 results to a client who perceives them as Level 3 results), the only thing an assessor can do is to try to successfully repair the relationship by acknowledging the blunder and role-modeling for the client how to deal with one's weaknesses and vulnerabilities. Attempting to repair "empathic disruptions" is said to be one of the best ways an assessor can build ego strength in clients. An analogy used by Finn (March 2009, personal communication) is that a Therapeutic Assessor's goal is to "midwife an insight" rather than "deliver a baby" at the end of the assessment. This makes perfect sense to me if the true goal is to have clients take ownership (and credit) for their self-discoveries. As therapists, we know that any new self-knowledge is bound to be significantly more meaningful if clients believe they have developed new insights into themselves through their own hard work of self-reflection and self-study.

## A CASE STUDY

A local Department of Social Services asked me to evaluate a 17-year-old woman who was brought on an emergency basis to one of their foster homes. Their goal was to get a psychologist's input on what kind of setting she should live in once the emergency placement expired and what, if any, clinical services would be needed to support her success in that environment. Thus, while their goal was primarily evaluative in nature, I was given implicit permission to approach the evaluation as a Therapeutic Assessment.

As I started the assessment, the only thing I knew about this young woman was that her extended family members could not take care of her and that she had been in 14 or 15 homes before this one. Immediately I hypothesized to myself that this person was suffering from Reactive Attachment Disorder and approached the assessment with this premise in mind.

The assessment process proved to be a humbling one for me, for as the data started coming in, my original hypothesis received less and less support. I learned that her extended family members could not care for her, not due to unmanageable behavior, but due to financial constraints. I learned that her multiple moves from home to home were, again, not attributable to behavior difficulties but circumstances beyond her control. I learned that she was suffering from numerous traumas that included not only various forms of abuse but death and abandonment by parent figures. I also learned to appreciate her genuine yearning for a sense of permanency in her life. Interestingly, her Rorschach data indicated that she possessed an accurate view of reality, exceedingly so at times, and that this contributed to her profound sadness and disappointment.

After explaining the original intent of the evaluation, I asked the young woman if she would like to generate questions that could satisfy curiosities about her own life. Within an hour, she developed seven questions! Four weeks later, I met with her, her therapist, and her most trusted child care worker to discuss the results, beginning the session with the question, "What is the worst thing I can tell you?" She quickly answered that I would recommend that she live with one particular family member. After reassuring her that I would not be making that recommendation, she relaxed and fully participated in the discussion, asking many questions and letting me know if the results were valid from her perspective. Shortly afterwards, I sent her a letter summarizing our session, excerpted below.

Dear Linda,*

I want to say thank you for allowing me into your life and giving me the privilege of getting to know you. You asked lots of good questions, and this letter is an attempt to summarize what we discussed the other night with your therapist. Before I do that, however, I want to say again how impressed I am with your ability to cope with the bad things that have gone on in your life. Some people who have been through what you have would have given up, and others may not have fared as well as you when it comes to controlling their behavior. In fact, one of your most effective coping mechanisms has been your ability to separate your thoughts and feelings about these events.

As you know, I tried to answer all seven of your questions. However, two of your questions could not be answered because I was unable to speak directly to your mother or father. In regard to your question about whether or not you would be able to have a relationship with either of your parents, the answer is that it would depend on *what kind* of relationship you desired. Remember, the word "responsibility" comes from "ability to respond." What you know now is that your parents are not able to respond to your needs and desires the way most parents are able to for their children. They have other challenges in life that prevent them from being as "responsible" as other parents are for their children and how you would like for them to be. The good news is that you have found ways to endear yourself to other adults who are very happy to have you depend on them, at least while you're a teenager. As you get older, you may find yourself depending on them as much as they depend on you, and that could feel very satisfying.

Your next set of questions has to do with why you feel forgotten or abandoned by other family members. The answer to these questions seems to be the same as the one above. For whatever reason, they are not able to respond to your needs. This reality hurts very deeply, I know. But please, remember, their "inability to respond" to your needs has nothing to do with you and your goodness as a person.

You asked why you've had to endure living in so many homes. I don't have a solid answer to that question but, as we discussed, the Chinese word for "crisis" is the same as "opportunity." Perhaps your moving from place to place has given you a unique perspective on life that will one day provide you with the opportunity to help others who find themselves in a similar kind of situation.

Finally, you asked "Why am I always smiling when I'm not happy?" This is probably the most challenging question of all. We talked about how "be-

*Name changed to protect confidentiality.

neath" your smiling face there is a huge amount of sadness from losing your mother and then, later, your aunt. We talked about how hard you try to not let anyone see your pain. Perhaps you are afraid of opening the floodgates, meaning that you are afraid that if you start to cry, you won't stop. Another possible reason is that you're afraid that if you don't show perfect behavior (and a smile), others might not accept you. To protect yourself, you have built up a very big, protective wall around your heart.

The question before you then, Linda, is whether you wish to do anything with these results and, if you do, how *fast* you want to do anything and *who* you want to help you with these changes. You are in charge. You can choose to keep things the way they are. Or you can choose to make some changes. When we met, you said you wanted to make some changes, like taking down the brick wall one brick at a time with the help of your therapist because you trust her.

Linda, as you know, I'm recommending to your caseworker that you have an opportunity to live with a therapeutic foster family. That means that the new family you live with will take you to your therapy sessions and participate in them whenever necessary in order for them to support you while you make these difficult but profoundly important personal changes.

With confidence that things will unfold for you the way that they should,

Dr. Rivera

## SUMMARY

In brief, a strengths-based approach to assessment is one way to affect positive change in a client's life. When this intent is combined with the implementation of a high-quality, collaborative approach to assessment, the results can be therapeutic. And when the results are shared in an ego-supportive manner, such as when following a Therapeutic Assessment protocol, the process can leave clients stronger, more empowered, more capable, more hopeful of change, and even more resilient in the face of challenges. In short, a humanistic approach to assessment—that is, bringing honor and reverence to our clients who permit themselves to be so vulnerable to us in the self-discovery process—can be both effective and ethically correct.

## REFERENCES

Finn, S. E. (2003). Therapeutic asessment of a man with "ADD." *Journal of Personality Assessment, 80*, 115–129.

Finn, S. E. (2007). *In our clients' shoes: Theory and techniques of therapeutic assessment.* Mahwah, NJ: Lawrence Ehrlbaum Associates.

Finn, S. E. & Tonsager, S. E. (1982). The therapeutic effects of providing MMPI-2 test feedback to college students awaiting psychotherapy. *Psychological Assessment: A Journal of Consulting and Clinical Psychology, 4*, 278–287.

Fischer, C. (1985/1994). *Individualizing psychological assessment.* Hillsdale, NJ: Lawrence Erlbaum Associates.

Handler, L. (2007). The use of therapeutic assessment with children and adolescents. In S. R. Smith & L. Handler (Eds.), *The clinical assessment of children and adolescents: A practitioner's handbook* (pp. 53–72). Mahwah, NJ: Lawrence Erlbaum.

Lance, B. R., & Krishnamurthy, R. (2003, March). A comparison of three modes of MMPI-2 test feedback. Paper presented at the annual meeting of the Society for Personality Assessment, San Francisco, CA.

Lerner, P. M. (2005). Red beavers and building bridges between assessment and treatment. *Journal of Personality Assessment, 85*(3), 271–279.

Newman, M. L., & Greenway, P. (1997). Assessment as a brief intervention. *Clinician's Research Digest, 15*(10), 1.

Satir, V., Banmen, J., Gerber, J., & Gomori, M. (1991). *The Satir model: Family therapy and beyond.* Palo Alto, CA: Science and Behavior Books, Inc.

Swann, W. B., Jr. (1996). *Self-traps: The elusive quest for higher self-esteem.* New York: Freeman.

Tharinger, D. J., Finn, S. E., Austin, C. A., Gentry, L. B., Bailey, K. E., Parton, V. T., & Fisher, M. E. (2008). Family sessions as part of child psychological assessment: Goals, techniques, clinical utility, and therapeutic value. *Journal of Personality Assessment, 90*(6), 547–558.

Tharinger, D. J., Finn, S. E., Hersh, B., Wilkinson, A., Christopher, G. B., & Tran, A. (2008). Assessment feedback with parents and preadolescent children: A collaborative approach. *Professional Psychology: Research and Practice, 39*(6), 600–609.

Tharinger, D. J., Finn, S. E., Wilkinson, A., DeHay, T., Parton, V. T., Bailey, K. E., & Tran, A. (2008). Providing psychological assessment feedback to children through individualized fables. *Professional Psychology: Research and Practice, 39*(6), 610–618.

Tharinger, D. J., Finn, S. E., Wilkinson, A. D., & Schaber, P. M. (2007). Therapeutic assessment with a child as a family intervention: A clinical and research case study. *Psychology in the Schools, 44*(3), 293–309.

White, M., & Epston, D. (1990). *Narrative means to therapeutic ends.* New York: W. W. Norton.

# 14

# Developing a Focus on Mental Health in the Head Start Classroom

*Andrew Fussner*

In a large federal effort to break the "cycle of poverty" the U.S. government established many programs to address the chronic impoverishment of many American families. As a part of the "War on Poverty" in 1965, President Lyndon Johnson proposed the creation of an educational program for young children from disadvantaged environments. Head Start was established with the intention to accomplish exactly what the name implies, that is, to give three-, four-, and five-year-old children from low-income areas an opportunity to get an early start in a school setting, which would give them the skills to succeed in elementary school. The first program in Head Start began as an eight-week summer session. Within a short period of time Head Start developed into a full-time, six-hours-per-day, five-days-per-week experience that offered children and families a range of services. Initiating an educational curriculum was just one part of the program. There was also the expectation that children enrolled in Head Start would be given social, emotional, psychological, and health services.

At this time there were numerous studies to determine the significance of the overall impact of the environment on the development of children, as well as methods of intervening. Urie Bronfenbrenner, a developmental psychologist at Cornell University, is regarded as "the father of Head Start." His long and distinguished career as an academic, researcher, and practitioner produced many contributions to the field of child development and educational environments. His studies of ecological systems theory resulted in his formulation of four types of systems. His paradigm included: (1) the microsystem, which is the family and classroom; (2) the mesosystem, which describes the interaction between the two microsystems; (3) the exosystem, which includes the external environments that influence the family and classroom; and (4) the macrosystem, which includes the larger social systems influencing all the systems.

Within the next several pages the interplay of the many systems that create the mental health environment in the Head Start classroom, and the many forces that influence the mental health of the three-, four-, and five-year-old child will be described. The mental health practitioner in the Head Start classroom needs several sets of lenses in order to get an accurate view of the child, the family, and the classroom. While appreciating the ecological systems theory of Professor Bronfenbrenner, multiple lenses will be provided to the practitioner including lenses to view the child, lenses to view the teacher and classroom, and lenses that focus on the child's family. The turning of a kaleidoscope of several lenses will allow the mental health practitioner to observe the many facets that contribute to the mental health of young children and to highlight the strengths of all the contributing systems.

## THE CHILD IN THE CLASSROOM

Tommy has been attending Head Start for the past four months. When he enters the classroom in the morning he eats his cereal by himself. He refuses to remove his coat. He never greets the teacher or her assistant in response to their saying good morning to him. After he finishes his cereal he throws the bowl and the milk carton into the basket and begins to wander around the classroom provoking other children. He takes their toys, drops books from the library corner onto the floor, takes a fistful of sand out of the sandbox and scatters it on the carpet. He pays no intention to the teachers who are inviting him to join them in an activity and stop his provocative behavior. After a few minutes of disruptiveness he seats himself in a far corner of the classroom and stares at the activities going on around him. He does not speak during these daily episodes.

In beginning a mental health consultation in a Head Start classroom, the consultant takes a focused view, as if using a spyglass to momentarily examine the child. In the course of the initial contact with a three-, four-, or five-year-old child, the consultant observes specific phenomenon that radiate from the child. These phenomena include the behavior, verbalizations, emotional tone, and appearances. The following is a description of areas that bring into focus the developmental achievements of the child and the qualities that make the child a unique person:

1. *The physical appearance of the child.* Does the child appear to be in good health and the expected size for his or her age? Does the child appear to be clean? Are his or her clothes clean? Is the impression on

first contact or observation of the child that there may be a delay in motor functioning or physical capabilities? If there are obvious delays in capacity or functioning upon first contact, it will be crucial to get a thorough developmental history.

2. *The language skills of the child.* There is a considerable range of developed skill in expressive language capacity among children ages three, four, and five. A three-year-old can usually speak in a sentence of a few words with a noun, verb, and perhaps another noun or an adjective. Some three-year-olds speak in several complete sentences. At five years there ought to be a clear capacity to string a few words together in a full sentence. Many four- and five-year-olds will tell stories with rich details and a wide range in vocabulary. In terms of receptive language the classroom staff will assure the mental health consultant the child seems to understand what the adults are communicating. As the school year progresses the routine of the classroom becomes very familiar to the children. It is considered best practice to have a routine every day with meal, toilet, circle time, play, structured activity, and so forth. After an initial period of adjustment the child should readily be able to follow the verbal directives of the teaching staff and demonstrate responsiveness to verbal suggestions that accompany the routine. It is very important that the consultant know which language is spoken in the home. In many Head Start classrooms, English is the second language to some children and may not be the spoken language in the home. If English is not spoken in the home it will be important to know about the child's capability in the family's language.
3. *Cognitive skills of the child.* Development in the area of cognitive skill is similar to the developmental trajectory of language in a young child. There is a wide range in children's capacity to learn in school. The expectations in Head Start include the child being able to identify letters, numbers, shapes, and colors. Some children learn easily at age three, other children require a longer period of time to understand and remember letters, numbers, and so forth. The vast majority of children are able to meet the expectations by the age of five. Many children are able to read before they enter kindergarten. The teaching staff is most often able to ascertain how the learning process is proceeding in each child. The mental health consultant is interested in knowing if and how the learning process is happening. Circle time in the morning, singing songs, and doing recitations at lunch time are all designed to build learning skills and to challenge the memory in the young child. It is essential for the mental health consultant to have a clear idea of how this learning process is developing.
4. *Attachments in the classroom.* Three-, four-, and five-year-old children have had relatively few important adults in their lives. These relationships

shape the nature of the child's attachment style. Most often the mother, father, grandmother, grandfather, aunt, uncle, and other family/community members are the significant others in the child's life. The family around the child has created a nest that nurtures and supports the child and teaches the child the method of forming attachments. For sure, each child is born with a specific temperament which influences his or her behavior and emotional vibration. The temperament of the child is understood by the significant family members or caretakers within the first few months of life. The family members accommodate the child's temperamental style and develop a rhythm which responds in harmony to the child. This responsiveness by the family members in conjunction with the child's temperament forms the basis for the child's attachment style. When children begin in Head Start they have an image of what to expect from an adult caregiver. This image is not made explicit by the children. They are not able to describe in words what they are expecting in relationships with adults. Instead the children enact their own expectations about relationships with caregivers. The mental health consultant inquires about the child's attachment to the teaching staff with the intention of understanding the child's attachment style. Does the child seem attached to the teaching staff? Does the child go to the teaching staff when he or she has a need or is upset? How does the child respond to words or gestures of recognition from the staff? Is the child able to accept comfort from the teaching staff? Teachers have many opportunities to observe family members in interaction with the child when the child is being accompanied to/from the classroom. What are the teachers' observations about the caretaker/child interaction? Some of the most dramatic and disturbing attachments are manifested by those young children who have had many disruptions in important relationships. Children who have been placed in several foster homes or who have been moved from one family member to another without continuity in relationships manifest the more problematic attachment style. Basic mistrust forms the foundation for the development of attachments in these young children, resulting in intense aggression or profound indifference toward the teaching staff. Children with traumatic attachment histories may exhibit poor boundaries with strangers. These children will become very friendly and needy in the presence of strangers, as if they are seeking an adult to take them home.

5. *Emotional expressiveness and regulation.* When children enter Head Start they are in most ways prepared to enjoy a full day in a classroom. They can walk, run, manually manipulate toys and objects, listen to stories with genuine curiosity, and engage other children in play. They are secure enough to leave the family nest for a few hours. The

emotional development of the child is at a delicate and fast-changing pace between the ages of three to five years. During the first few years of life the emotional state of the child has dominated his or her consciousness, and the emotional needs of the child have held center stage in driving the child toward others and toward various activities. As a standard part of the Head Start curriculum the emotional capacities of the child are challenged in two ways. The child is given many opportunities to learn to identify the range of feelings he or she may be experiencing. Being able to identify and express these feelings is an important developmental milestone for the child during the Head Start experience. "I feel sad," "I feel angry," "I am happy." "The child in the story is feeling happy." These identifications and expressions are crucial for a child to begin to develop skill in understanding himself or herself. Many classrooms have posters hanging on the wall that illustrate faces with specific emotions on them. There are many storybooks which illustrate children attempting to identify and express emotions. As children accomplish expressive skill in relation to their own feelings they will then begin to develop mastery over the emotions. Achieving some mastery over the driving force of emotions and utilizing language to express emotions fosters the quick acceleration of thinking capacity in the child. In infants and toddlers there is almost no differentiation between feeling/fantasy and action. A three- or four-year-old child will develop the skill in expressing his or her emotions and in so doing will experience the emergence of thinking as an intermediary between feeling/fantasy and action. The mental health consultant appreciates that these skills of identifying and expressing emotions, and beginning to think about oneself and one's own emotions are emerging during the Head Start years and will continue to strengthen over the course of childhood. It is the initial emergence of these skills which is important to the child at this stage in his or her development. Mastery of these skills takes much longer.

6. *Play*. Play is work. Play is an experiment. Play generates meaning. These are the concepts that are the most useful in observing and understanding a young child's play. The classroom offers many opportunities and choices for the child. Each classroom has brief periods during the day when the child can select a specific area or activity to engage in free or open play. Which activity or area the child selects has meaning for the child. When the child engages in play there is a mixture of fantasy and action that becomes illuminated to the observer. The child has selected this particular activity because it represents an issue that warrants further exploration by the child. The child could be attempting to develop a better understanding of a situation in his or her own life. The child could be testing his or her own capacity to

master an activity or situation. For example, the sandbox may involve the filling up and emptying of a container (the feeling of being filled with the presence of another and then the feeling of being absent from the other); the dinosaurs may involve fighting, eating each other, or getting into a straight line (the power of aggression or the ordering of aggression); the dress-up corner (the possibility of being another or the possibility of being a grown-up); the kitchen may involve preparing dinner or telling others what to do (the act of feeding or being fed, the act of nurturing or being nurtured). The playground, the reading area, the computer table, the shelves filled with blocks, and many more corners in the classroom represent possibilities for the child to explore, enact, or understand an emerging issue. For the observer/consultant, play is the symbolic mythology the child is generating to communicate to others the forces that are moving through his or her reality at this time.

8. *Socialization.* Head Start gives the child the opportunity to socialize with other children and adults. In most situations the child's socialization has been with family members or familiar caretakers. Children learn socialization skills from the moment they display the first smile at the arrival of a familiar face; generally in the third month of life. From that moment onward the child will have many interactive encounters with others and will begin to acquire more complex socialization skills. During the toddler years children play alongside other children, often referred to as "parallel play," but do not engage in a back and forth interaction. The Head Start experience gives the child a large network of new persons, both adults and peers, to test and expand the socialization skills they have already acquired. Most children in Head Start engage in a mixture of at times parallel, at other times interactive play. As the child grows from three to five years old they will engage in more interactive play and receive additional pleasure and ideas from the connection with peers. The mental health consultant observes how the child engages with other children, whether the child has shown an interest in particular peers, and whether at times the child seeks the involvement of a peer. The child who has been attending Head Start for a few weeks can recite the names of some of his or her friends in the classroom. Most children continue to enjoy playing alone at times. Indeed, the need to be alone with oneself hardly ever disappears throughout life. Children in Head Start will consistently exhibit a mixture of self-play and social play. The mental health consultant will, however, have a heightened concern for the child who demonstrates no interest or no skill in engaging peers. The presence of adults in the classroom also offers an opportunity for the child to demonstrate his capacity, style,

and skill in engaging grown-ups. As there are many different families there are many different styles of engagement displayed by children when they venture out into the world and reproduce the method of making a connection with adults that they have learned at home. Children show a preference for certain adults. It is common that a child will prefer the teacher to the assistant teacher, or prefer the assistant to the teacher. There are many possible interpretations for this occurrence but what is more significant is whether the child engages at all. The consultant is interested in the child's receptivity to warmth, concern, affection, correction, and discipline as it occurs between the child and adults in the classroom.

## THE TEACHER AND THE CLASSROOM

Ms. Roberts calls out to Tommy and offers him the possibility to play the drums or the horn with two other boys in the music corner. Tommy behaves as if he does not hear her. Ms. Roberts turns her attention to other children in the room, at which point Tommy escalates his behavior by picking up another child's truck and walking away with it, leading a crying, protesting peer on a chase toward the back corner of the classroom. Shamir, the boy whose truck was taken, is clearly angry, and has no intention of letting Tommy get away with this theft in broad daylight.

Ms. Roberts walks briskly across the room toward the boys while calling out to Tommy the rules of sharing and not taking things without asking permission. He quickly eludes her and moves with the truck above his head toward the play kitchen area where the other children are stopping their free play and beginning to observe the chase. Ms. Roberts is closing in on Tommy. Her assistant screams out to Tommy, "I am calling your mother right now! I am not putting up with another day of your bad behavior." Ms. Roberts says to her assistant, "Let me handle this for now." Shamir, in pursuit of Tommy the truck thief, has accidentally knocked over the tea party arrangement that Marisa and Jamie had set up for their friends. Marisa begins to cry. Ms. Roberts realizes she has less than 60 seconds to avoid a deluge.

The Head Start classroom is most often the first classroom experience for the child. In order to grasp the significance and range of this experience the consultant/observer will need to utilize binocular lenses. In using the binocular lenses the consultant can broaden the view to examine the entire field as well as at times focus in on a particular feature of the setting. Head Start is a full day of activity and expectation beginning at 8:45 a.m. and ending at 3 p.m. There are 15 or more children in each class with two adult teachers who are responsible to provide for the children and offer an educational curriculum. The children depend on the teachers for a wide range of their needs. Recognition when they do a good job, help when they become frustrated in a task, guidance through challenges with other children, giving them new social skills, introducing new words to aid in expressing feelings, opening the hot containers at lunch time, helping when there has been an accident in the toilet, settling onto the cots at nap time are a few of the thousands of needs the teachers will face in an ordinary week in the classroom. In addition to the social and emotional instructions the teachers are expected to teach the children letters, numbers, colors, calendars, songs, seasons, and scores of other important educational skills. This is an impossible task for any ordinary human being. This is an impossible task for any extraordinary human being. In understanding the mental health features of a Head Start classroom it is crucial that the consultant/observer appreciates the stressful nature of working with young children hour after hour, day after day, week after week with the added complexity of variations in health, weather, and familial circumstance in the lives of the children and the teachers. To be the sole two adults in the classroom for 15 or more children is a very draining experience.

An often underappreciated aspect of the Head Start environment is the exceptional emotional closeness that develops between the teachers and the children; that is, how very much the teacher begins to take on the parental/caretaker/guardian role toward the children in her classroom. This identificatory process is most often unconscious but its appearance is inevitable when so many young children are placed under the protective umbrella of an adult and the adult automatically responds to the challenge. There are moments when teachers are extremely frustrated and lack patience with a particular child or several children. Underlying these negative emotions, the deep protective impulses of the adult continue to be active and influential. "These are my children"; "My child is not behaving properly" are two refrains playing in the mind of the teacher simultaneously with her complaints. It is this phenomenon which necessitates the consultant to adopt a strengths-based, respectful, and empowering attitude toward the teachers. During the course of a school year a special rhythm develops between the teacher and each child such that the teacher knows the soul and the mind of each child and is able to engage or respond to each child in the unique manner that fits that particular child. It is the achievement of this rhythm that creates the holding environment which allows learning and growth to emerge and prosper in each child.

The teacher is a human being. The teacher is asked to create the most warm and functional holding environment for the children. Who takes care of the teacher? How is the context around the teacher and her staff? The teacher needs to feed the children. Who is feeding the teacher? They show reverence for the children, who shows reverence for the teachers?

The mental health consultant will inquire about these matters in a discreet and respectful manner. Since the beginning of time it has been understood that the well-being of the parent or guardian will affect the well-being of the children. The same idea applies to the classroom. One area of inquiry for the consultant is the relationship between the teacher and her staff. After a few hours in the classroom, as the daily schedule unfolds and the various activities are completed, the nature of the relationship between the teacher and her staff begins to emerge for the consultant/observer. The consultant observes the synchrony of a pitcher and a catcher, of a two-person singing duet, of two people who know each other well enough to be able to predict the thoughts and moves of the other, of two persons who know their individual differences and can create a balance that works for both of them. The relationship contains the capability of the sharing of affection, frustration, joy, humor, sadness, irony, and the rolling of eyes toward the heavens in a communication of "can you believe this one." Because the Head Start classroom is an emotionally difficult and draining setting, the teacher and staff need to be cared for and have the experience that they will be able to turn to another when there is a need or when the tide of immaturity is rising too high. If the classroom setting is lacking in support for the staff or if the relationship between the teacher and her assistant is unsupportive, it is likely the essential immaturity of the context will overwhelm the adults and the emotional tone of the classroom will stabilize at the developmental stage of early childhood.

The teacher is an employee. Many Head Start programs are housed in schools or agencies that have the classrooms as a part of a wider mission in the community. The employees are responsible to the administration of the school or agency. There is also a supervisory structure that is situated within the program. The teaching staff in the Head Start classroom is employed within a wider system that can have a powerful effect on the atmosphere of the classroom. A mental health consultant would always be curious about the familial context of the client in a psychotherapy setting. The same idea holds true for the consultant entering into a classroom. What is the relationship between the classroom staff and the agency? How supported or how neglected is the staff of the classroom?

The teacher is a daughter. The teacher may be a mother. The teacher has a family life that resonates within her. Teachers, psychotherapists, social workers, physicians, and other professions that require the engagement of another person on a personal level may activate the histories or current stories that contribute to a particular interpersonal style. When the teacher is standing in front of the class or seated on her stool reading to the children at circle time her history as a child, her memories of her parents, her current relationships are in the room with her. The consultant realizes that those stories from the past or current conflictual relationships may possibly contribute to the development of problematic connections with the children or staff in the classroom. In a most delicate and respectful manner, after a trusting relationship has developed between the consultant and the teacher, it is appropriate for the consultant to inquire "Is it OK if I ask you some questions about yourself?"

## THE FAMILY OF THE CHILD

Ms. Wilson, Tommy's mother, leaves her job as a technician at the local community hospital everyday at 2:30 p.m. She promptly enters the classroom at 3 p.m., helps Tommy gather his coat, his daily projects, the note to parents, and his sleeping bear. She then looks to Ms. Roberts for the nod of "good day" or "bad day" that is communicated in the slightest tilt of the head. On this afternoon Ms. Roberts gestures to Ms. Wilson for a brief conversation about the events of a roller-coaster day for her son. Tommy senses the vibrations between the adults. He holds his sleeping bear near the side of his face as his teacher and mother speak to each other. When the two adults have finished speaking Ms. Wilson takes Tommy by the hand and walks out of the classroom without saying a word to him. Tommy looks at his mother's face while pretending not to look. He can see the tears in her eyes and feel the tightness in her grip of his hand. They walk together in silence out of the school building.

The family is the most important context for young children. It is primarily within the family context that the young child learns the most significant emotional and interpersonal lessons for life. It is primarily within the family context that the child learns his or her own sense of self. When children enter the Head Start classroom they display their family and the family's history and culture. Perhaps not as obvious as a sleeping bear or a photo of a new puppy, the family nonetheless arrives each day in the classroom in the way the child presents his or her own sense of self and in the interpersonal style of the child. The mental health consultant in the Head Start classroom gathers as much information as possible about the child's family context. Who lives in the home? Who cares for the child? How are the caretaking roles distributed among the various family members? With whom is the child most close? To whom does the child turn in moments of distress or inquiry? Does the child spend parts of the week in one home and parts in another setting? In developing a workable hypothesis for understanding a child's emotional state or behavioral repertoire the consultant develops a map of the family structure that includes all the interpersonal arrangements of the significant persons in the child's life at this time. The map of the family relationships illustrates for the consultant the quality of closeness and distance among the family members, the emotional circuitry, the expressed and unexpressed affective tones. Historical information about the family also places the family in its own context and deepens the understanding of current themes and struggles that may be occurring. Trauma, divorce, marital separation, loss through death or illness, episodes of abuse, and lack of basic financial resources are a few of the events in the history and the situation of a family that may impact the current structure and quality of the relationships. The most important feature in developing an understanding of the family is the fact that young children, ages three, four, and five years old, are not well differentiated from their caretakers. If there is distress in the lives of the caretakers the child will feel it. He or she will not often talk about it because the topic is very distressing to the child and the caretaker. Silence on the part of the child is very often a gesture of protection toward the caretaker. The child holds the emotion and houses the memory while simultaneously constructing an explanation which is more often than not an immature, inaccurate one.

The consultant inquires about the well-being of the parents or caretakers. The consultant needs to become comfortable in asking questions of the adults in the child's life. If the family is convinced that the consultant is confident that such information is important they will be forthcoming with responses. In working with Head Start families many parents and caretakers do not appreciate how much young children observe and how deeply they are affected by the emotional states of their loved ones. "Oh, he is always playing"; "He doesn't really know what is going on"—common expressions that are commonly untrue. "Is it OK if I ask you a few questions about yourself?" "In order to help me better understand your child it would be useful for me to ask you a few questions," is one way for the consultant to expand the view of the child and to introduce into the perspective an understanding of the processes in the context.

Every parent has a life. Whether it is as an employee, spouse, student, manager, technician, choir member, volunteer, daughter, granddaughter, or grandmother, the parent or caretaker performs multiple roles and is subjected to many different demands in daily life. These roles, if productive and satisfying, sustain the rich sense of self the parent harbors. Maintaining that rich sense of self is important to the young child who is living in the same nest. The most accurate view of the child includes a view of the family context and a clear understanding of the relationships within the family.

## TOMMY IN ACTION: TOMMY IN CONTEXT

*Tommy*. His behavior demonstrates that he does not want to be in school today. He chooses to be by himself. A child who typically does socialize may avoid other children or adults on a particular day because he is attempting to avoid certain feelings that are too upsetting to identify or express at this time. On this day Tommy has arrived in school with some conflictual issue brewing inside which likely originated at home. Tommy is eating by himself with his coat buttoned and not interested in taking it off. He is not getting comfortable with staying in class today. He is eating. He is sitting at the table. It is useful to look at what the child is doing that is functional at this moment. During the difficult moment of a child's acting out, the staff frequently overlooks the adaptive efforts the child is making. The intensity of the acting out dominates the scenario, and the perspective of the staff becomes narrower. As Tommy moves around the classroom he provokes his peers and draws them into conflict with him and creates a disturbance for the teacher and her assistant. Does the sight of other children playing with each other stimulate jealousy in Tommy? Does he select to grab the truck from his peer because the peer has something that Tommy does not have at this time? Is there an old grudge between the two boys? Does he wander indiscriminately among his peers hoping to provoke them all and make them all angry with him? Is he wishing to be rejected by everyone at this time? He holds the truck above his head and struts around the room possibly imagining he is a truck driver and getting on the highway and going far away from this moment. When he goes to the seat and isolates himself and sits in silence, what is he thinking? Why does he select the silent sitting at this moment? In children of Head Start–age, fantasy and action are opposite sides of the same coin. There is a narrative being played out in his mind at this time and it is best for the consultant to try to ascertain the content of that narrative before beginning to make an intervention. The consultant imagines being the child for the next few minutes, plays the scenario as if it were a script in a theater piece and the consultant attempts to grasp what the playwright is hoping to communicate.

The teacher will want to intervene with Tommy as soon as possible. She can see that he is escalating his behavior and beginning to create a disturbance among the other children. The domino effect in which one child's behavior gets quickly replicated in another child is quite common in Head Start. Another child might become frightened of Tommy's behavior or become afraid that he or she will be overcome with their own aggression and create some havoc with other children. Defenses against powerful emotions are not firmly established at this age; sometimes a small amount of stimulation leads to an eruption. The teacher in this instance will try to get as close as possible to Tommy. Sitting with him and most likely holding his hand or having some physical contact with him will aid the engagement of the child. "I can sense that you are upset this morning," "I could see when you came in this morning you had something on your mind." "I do not know what is on your mind . . . perhaps something happened at home this morning . . . or you were remembering something . . . or someone said something to you. . . ." The strategy consists of the teacher putting into words possibilities for the child. The teacher is striving to offer some words to Tommy and invite him to engage in a two-step process: (1) put a word or words on his feelings/memories/fears at this moment; (2) express in a sentence what it is/was that may be on his mind and spilling out into his morning in the classroom. "You are a good boy and I can help you put into words whatever it is that is bothering you. . . . Once you put it into words you will not feel so upset and you will enjoy your morning in the classroom." The teacher shows curiosity, not certainty, about what may be troubling Tommy, and she invites him to verbalize rather act out. Tommy, as many children do, might say he does not know what is bothering him. The teacher accepts his uncertainty and offers to have a once-every-10-minutes check-in with her. "Once every 10 minutes I will quietly speak to you and ask you how you are feeling." "You and I together can work on this troubling feeling and place words on it so you do not need to misbehave when these feelings erupt again."

The most ideal intervention includes the family members beginning to help Tommy express in words those troubling emotions which he is afraid might overwhelm him and those persons who are close to him. In speaking with the mother at the end of the day, the teacher or the consultant will tell her the events of the morning and help her to understand that there is an opportunity here for Tommy to grow in his expressive capabilities. It will be helpful to Tommy if his parents or caretakers can also begin to help him, teach him, and to explore with him any worries or sadnesses that he might have this time. The best therapeutic scenario includes the family and the teaching staff working together in creating a helpful atmosphere for Tommy. The best relationship between teacher, family, and consultant includes the recognition that the mother herself appears to be stressed at times, and the offer to meet with her.

Tommy's presentation in the classroom is illustrative of one among thousands of possible behavioral possibilities in the Head Start setting. The mental health consultant performs best practice by using a kaleidoscope of images, allowing the child, the teacher, and the classroom contexts to move interchangeably in formulating a clinical perspective and a plan for intervention. Reverence for the child, reverence for the family, and reverence for the teacher, they deserve no less.

# 15

# What's "Good for the Goose": The Strengths-Based Approach with Providers

*Susan Cristantiello and Andrew Kuntz*

In the interest of immediate and full disclosure, the authors admit to being ringers—well, actually, we like to think we're each other's ringers or pinch-hitters. We have had a personal and professional relationship for over 30 years, which includes receiving our core training in the same graduate program. We have had ample opportunity to support each other's development and reflect each other's professional growth in our work, and to act as sounding boards for each other's practice. We count ourselves very fortunate. However, to the point of this chapter, we function in roles at Astor Services for Children and Families in Dutchess and Bronx Counties in New York that speak to the heart of our thesis, as the program director of an urban children's outpatient mental health clinic and the supervisor of Coordinated Children's Services Initiative (CCSI), a community-based services program that is entirely focused on supporting strengths and resiliencies of children and families.

It would be both a truth and a generalization to say that one of us has been deficit-focused with regard to our professional outlook and practice, while the other has been strengths-based. The "truth" of the statement is that these are the poles around which our types of programs have traditionally orbited, while the generalization is that we have mitigated one another's point of view with a profound appreciation for work of the other. Further, we have been supported by our agency in modifying and amending traditional programmatic points of view. And, as long as we're being completely candid, the shared influence is not equal, for the clinic director has absorbed a greater measure of professional change from the community service coordinator.

This is the thesis for our chapter: strengths-based approaches in work with children and families not only provide a process model that can be effectively integrated into clinical treatment, but also provide a parallel-process model for helping groups composed of care providers be more effective in recognizing and responding to resilient features of children and families.

The mental health field has been gradually evolving from a deficit-based focus that is notoriously centered on pathology, toward a strengths and prevention model, albeit in a very gradual reorientation (Allison, 2003). This process began with identification of biases and politicization in identification and categorization of deficits in client presentations. For example, much has been written over the past several decades about biases that contribute to "pathologizing" phenomenon, even characterizing psychiatric diagnosis as an "essentially political enterprise of naming psychological distress" (Morris, 1997). Similarly, accusations of "over-pathologizing" of individuals come from several points of view, not infrequently used to support a political agenda. Such "over-pathologizing" has been described from the standpoint of race and ethnicity, gender (Morris, 1997), age, cognitive ability, and so on—and not without merit in many cases, for there are indeed documented excesses of each in the historical record of general psychiatric practice. Within memory, for example, is the de-pathologizing of homosexuality, dropped from the DSM II in 1974, and the dubious inclusion of PMDD (severe PMS) in 1994.

Jean Campbell (1998) reviewed the literature on consumerism, outcomes, and satisfaction and concluded: "Traditional mental health systems pathologize problems in living, hold low expectations of consumer achievement, are paternalistic, offer a limited range of options, and define anger as symptomatic. Key concerns included the threat of involuntary treatments, subtle forms of coercion, lack of respect toward consumers by mental health professionals and providers, and the debilitating side-effects of medications . . . researchers fail to ask questions that would capture the detrimental effects of treatment and care" (p. 21). Furthermore, "controlling symptoms and behavior of consumers and maintaining the effectiveness of the service system are expressed priorities of mental health professionals, while consumers ask, 'What does this do for my life?'" (p. 21).

Concurrent with criticism of the traditional deficit-focused models of treatment, there have been increased attention on the effects of resiliency, popularly thought of as the capacity to rebound from adversity. A Division 29 APA Task Force convened in 2001 to investigate factors that resulted in positive outcomes in psychotherapy, chaired by John Norcross, determined that some 40 percent of successful outcomes were attributable to patient characteristics, among which resiliency was a primary factor (Norcross, 2002). The writers believe that resiliency is also a useful and perhaps underestimated factor in effective teamwork, as will be explained. Michael Rutter

(1999) concluded that a range of factors impact a typical presentation in therapy and that both protective and risk factors are equally impacted, and thus attention should be paid to both. Resilience, writes Rutter, "does not constitute an individual trait or characteristic" (p. 135). Instead, children demonstrate and practice resilience in different social situations, thus increasing the protective aspects for life's later challenges. Providers too practice resilience in work situations. Team and family meetings, home visits, community meetings, all challenge us in different ways and therefore call upon a repertoire of resilience.

Professional training and identity for mental health professionals and mental health systems continues to stress the application of active interventions in the face of assessed deficits. Procedures that are prescriptive and intrusive seem to be as prevalent as collaborative processes that target resiliency; far too often, treatment staff believe themselves responsible for the burden of alleviating through their direct action a palliative response to client distress. Professionals typically believe they must produce a direct effect, "craft an intervention" and to "prescribe" when faced with dysfunction. Similarly, treatment programs are sculpted to "apply remedies" in an organized fashion. Perhaps this accounts for the plethora of "dis-" words in our professional conversation: dysfunction, dysregulation, distress, dystonia, distortion, and so on—how odd the same nonprefixed words sound (and how insightfully alienated youth complain of being "diss'd"). Language, it has been pointed out, is a profound tool in shaping our perceptions and critical thinking about a phenomenon.

Family therapist William Madsen (2007c) calls such personal and professional phenomenon "inadvertent disempowering processes" and challenges professionals to recognize such practices, to understand how they position us in particular relationships with our colleagues, and to rethink how to act. Madsen finds these disempowering processes to be embedded in many of our professional discourses, in which "presumed truths" are often at the core of interaction. Presumed truths are the "value of professional expertise" versus collaboration, the focus on deficits rather than possibilities, and "professional responsibilities to clients based on paternalism" rather than accountability. Discourses based on presumed truths, Madsen states, "are often prescriptive, and include cultural specifications about how people should be and against which people compare themselves. They both reflect the prevailing social and political structures and tend to support them" (p. 5).

Presumed truths are frequently found to insert themselves in meetings of people with varying points of view, even of well-meaning provider groups in our experience. For example, at a recent discharge planning collaboration a provider asked a mother in an abusive relationship to explain to her husband (the absent abuser), instructing her in specific language to use, so that he would be amenable to the services. The mother looked at the community worker and could find no words. The presumed truth is that mothers are responsible for the behaviors and failures of all family members. The facilitator intervened, clearly stating that we understood she was not responsible for her husband's connection to the service provider. Her eyes welled up and she turned to the community worker with renewed confidence. He asked if it wouldn't be better if he called her husband and spoke to him directly. She countered with an invitation for him to come to the home to meet her husband. The community worker agreed readily, as this was the nature of his service. Most providers, when alerted to the pitfalls of stereotype and bias, will attempt to disabuse themselves of such misconceptions. The example is an important one because it is overwhelmingly the mother who interfaces with her children's providers, and who is often misrepresented as the only responsible party. The writers believe it is not just an individual task for each provider to wrestle with, but a collective endeavor so that we all may benefit from each other's vigilance.

Concurrent with the shift from deficit-based thinking to strengths-based approaches is the deinstitutionalizing of mental health. To reduce the need for costly residential and milieu treatment, networks of support services are required to sustain functioning in the community. Some treatment models have directly targeted this need and a number of systemic treatments have become prominent, and indeed "collaborative treatment" has become a current catchphrase for supportive programming. In use within Astor clinical programs are the collaborative evidence-based practices of Trauma Systems Therapy (Saxe, Ellis, & Kaplow, 2007) and Collaborative Problem Solving (Greene & Ablon, 2005). These and similar procedures have been devised specifically to help stabilize and improve functioning levels of individuals through the actions of a team of responders—professional and nonprofessional—to help intervene by matching needs with service providers. Each has developed, or is in the process of compiling, an evidence base to underpin their successful treatment strategies, and, anecdotally, we have found each to be effective in clinical application with children and families. The mental health professional need not spearhead such systems interventions, and there is room to argue that they should not be. Glen Saxe, B. Heidi Ellis, and Julie Kaplow (2007), for example, believe that TST teams (which include at minimum a home-based component, a legal advocate, a psychiatrist, and a therapist) can be successfully coordinated by any member of the team, professional or nonprofessional, who is willing and able to serve in the coordinating capacity.

The operant word "collaborative" has a multiplicity of meanings, however, depending upon one's point of view. In our experience "collaborative treatment" often unfortunately means that mental health professionals collaborate with one another, and only incidentally with consumers, to form care plans and support systems—it is the procedure that is collaborated on. The child and family often are only the recipients of the plan, and yet are expected to respond to it and carry it through as "received wisdom." We much prefer the process-focused concepts of collaboration outlined by Madsen in which the child and family are integral and equal partners in solving a problem. As Narrative Therapy proscribes, the child/family are seen as being in a relationship with a problem rather than being a problem, and thus partnerships can be formed between them and the support systems that "taps the resourcefulness of both." Madsen (2007b) proposes that helpers cultivate a preferred relational stance of an "appreciative ally" with the child/family, grounded in "respect, connection, curiosity and hope," in which the supporting system is experienced by the client as being "in their corner" or "on their side" (p. 22).

No Astor Services for Children and Families program embraces these concepts more fully than does the Coordinated Children's Service Initiative (CCSI). Referrals are made to the program when a child is at risk of removal from their home, and when they are involved in two or more service systems (e.g., mental health, probation, Department of Social Services, special education). The child and family are interviewed at home to allow them to share their concerns and strengths in a comfortable environment. CCSI then attempts to locate resources in their community that address those concerns and that build strengths shared in the interview. Once resources are located, the family, their current providers, and key representatives of the new sources are invited to a network meeting. The purpose of the meeting is for the family to devise a plan of action, using any combination of services present or suggested by the group in accordance with the wishes of the child and family. This purpose is not new, nor the method original, but some features are unique. First, the most vocal person in the meeting is the child, who is spoken "with," not "about." Second, participants may not be from the traditional "helping" or social service professions but may be representatives of various entities typically found in any community—police gang experts, employment agencies, mediators, coaches, clergy, and so on. Third, the family dictates the final plan of action rather than being the recipient of a prefashioned plan. Certainly, timely suggestions of the group are solicited, but so are those of the child. Fourth, participants are asked to think and respond beyond their professional expertise and narrow foci of their agencies and offer possible connections using their own strengths: personal areas of interest, knowledge of the neighborhood, and experience.

It is the network facilitator's job to make sure the communication remains appropriate and tailored to the stated concerns of the child and family, yet allow participants to be spontaneous. This eclectic mix of adults brings with them different approaches and philosophies but also present divergent and sometimes cross-purposes. They have varying inclinations to talk, potential biases, and differing levels of tolerance for meetings. They are subject to time constraints, are often overworked, and may be wary about being subjected to any additional vicarious traumatization from hearing more sad stories. Furthermore, they are asked to remove themselves from the comfort zone of reliance on their individual professional roles and instead are invited to share as equals, revealing something of themselves apart from agency description and title.

What motivates such a diverse group and supplies the potential for effectiveness? We think it is the same phenomenon that Norcross (2002) and the APA Task Force determined made individual clinical sessions effective—an approach that taps individual strengths and resiliencies, and values the often hidden talents of its participants. The facilitator alone is not required to be the "charismatic adult" described in the literature of resilience—it helps—but must allow the child to shine with all the charisma they posses, and must, in turn, allow the providers to shine in the eyes of the child. When providers are free from the responsibility to solve one problem—the problem their agency provides services for—they stop trying to fit the child's statements into a particular niche. They are free to listen to everything because the focus is broad. The whole child, the whole family, indeed the whole neighborhood is being addressed.

A detective attending a network once flipped out his notepad, "Columbo-style," and immediately began scribbling everything the child said in response to his question. When the facilitator explained that she would jot down on the board any relevant facts the family agreed to share and that he would get a copy, he acknowledged his occupational instinct, laughed, and admitted he was glad he could relax. He then refocused his attention on the child and away from his notepad and familiar agenda. As providers we were charmed by his guilelessness. The child, removed from being an object of observation, enjoyed the chance to talk to an authority figure as an equal member of this gathering.

In a comfortable atmosphere where our professions are not the starring roles we can concentrate on what we share—concern for children, and when we are not required to solve one problem in our field of expertise we are open to a world of possibilities and broader connections that are necessary for creative problem solving. It is one of the many contradictions tolerated and enjoyed in such a meeting. The child is asked to share as the expert—the only one in possession of their whole truth. In a typical network meeting there might be a therapist, youth service provider, guidance counselor, child protective worker, photo teacher, movement therapist, and director of a community center, all present at the same table. We never know who it will be that forms the leading edge of insight into a child's situation or the one who will inspire that child. Sometimes people are present without ever uttering a word, and are allowed the luxury of listening. A silent teacher at a meeting may be a valuable asset because the child is now convinced something different is going on, and it is this "difference" that captures their real attention. When grown-ups are not behaving predictably (boring, intimidating, hard-to-understand, not really interested in a child's opinion) they become fascinating creatures, are easier to talk to, and can become valuable friends.

A child protective worker from the local Department of Social Services, a stylish woman, offered knowledge of a secondhand boutique in the area that sold trendy and affordable clothing. This appealed to a teen who had just shared her reluctance to attend school, for one reason, because of her less than fashionable hand-me-downs. Seemingly simple exchanges like this one are valued for the empathic connections made as well as the information provided.

When individual colleagues expose strengths that may have been heretofore untapped it transforms into group strength where all members become equally free to try something different. As Montagu Don (1997) remarks in his book *The Sensuous Garden*, "To see the world as a child sees it, or as Van Gogh or William Blake saw it, we must be prepared to unlearn, to let go of the baggage of knowledge and respond to instinct" (p. 31). Relaxed providers are less defended, competitive, and single-minded. They let their minds wander over boundaries and in so doing discover themselves in interesting places. A youth service worker relates to the drumming interests of a child; a probation officer shares the address of a yoga center for meditation classes the child is seeking; and a respite coordinator passes on a phone contact from her sister-in-law, the college admissions advisor. The serious-faced principal makes a joke that may diffuse tension better than if it had come from a witty colleague, the more impactful because it was unexpected. Charming detectives, quiet instructors—what is going on? We are becoming appreciative allies, not of the child this time but of one another. We believe this process epitomizes the "coresearch" that Madsen describes as the ideal process of collaborative inquiry in individual and family treatment.

We have asked ourselves how do we influence systems of care—which often act in ways risk averse and controlling, self-perpetuating, paternalizing, with low expectations of consumer achievement—to shift their relational stances? We have found that working effectively with such systems in a strengths-based and proactive way entails a great deal of parallel process. Clients in individual therapy may present defensively, be ambivalent about taking risks, and have harmful personal scripts. A strengths-based treatment would entail identifying competencies, supporting their use and promoting their development, along with supportive cognitive reframing to support shifts in self-perception. When sufficient resources have been built up, the individual is encouraged and gently challenged to practice new behaviors. So, too, do we influence systems that seek to care for clients.

**Table 15.1**

| *Tenets of Strengths-Based Approach with Children* | Corollary Use with Providers |
|---|---|
| "The availability of alternative positive perceptions of themselves" | When providers view themselves in a holistic way, they have access to a range of self-perceptions that may allow them to connect to a wider range of people.<br><br>When a child asked, "If I take a pill for my ADHD will I stop being my crazy self? I like my crazy self." A provider, who had been quite vocal and self-revealing, responded: "Do I seem crazy to you or just plain regular?" "Crazy!" the child replied happily. "Well, I take pills for ADHD too. It didn't change me, just gave me extra powers to focus on things I want to—like you. Oh, and I don't get in as much trouble as I used to," she smiled. The child approached the provider in a serious way at the end of the meeting to continue a discussion of the effects of medication. |
| "Parents/caregivers who have developed their own sense of resilience to stress and provide this as a model" | In the network meeting providers are sometimes faced with frustrating conundrums and heart-wrenching situations. In response to this they each demonstrate their own brand of resilience. A provider simply pauses and all see how silence is sometimes the best offering. Someone else makes a tender remark and we see how an expression of true feeling can be appropriate, not patronizing. Someone else makes a witty observation and we see that it is OK to smile in the midst of pain. When these are offered in a spontaneous and genuine way the whole group experiences reinforced resilience. |
| "The encouragement given to develop positive relationships with other people, particularly caring and knowledgeable adults who are physically and emotionally available" | When members leave a collaborative meeting with stronger working ties than before, their relationship grows beyond the family that brought them together. We have often seen providers who have been to one meeting continue to call on one another for a variety of other collaborations. Caregivers are reminded that they have the same need as those they serve for relationships that sustain them in their work and personal development. |
| "The provision of consistency, predictability, structure, and clear expectations and boundaries in educational or recreational programs" | Providers, too, need to count on fellow agencies for consistent philosophy and procedure, so they know whom to turn to for what. Clear expectations and boundaries are necessary to keep the network meetings focused on the goal of connecting the family to resources and not exposing them to the scrutiny of multiple providers. A school psychologist, unfamiliar |

| *Tenets of Strengths-Based Approach with Children* | Corollary Use with Providers |
|---|---|
| | with the network process, began to delve into the child's diagnosis with the parent, resulting in the child's withdrawal and the parent becoming visibly upset. This may have been appropriate in another setting. The facilitator redirected the process by restating the goals of network and the family reengaged with the group. |
| "The opportunity for emotional expression in safe ways and places (i.e., to tell their stories and be listened to)" | Regardless of their social/emotional style, providers, like family members, are made to feel that their contributions will be welcomed.<br>At times the network table is allowed to be a melee of controlled chaos when participants are charged with the energy of addressing a particular concern. This is only safe and effective because the facilitator remains in her role as a conductor of a powerful ensemble. |

*Source*: Left-hand column was adapted from Allison et al. (2003) pp. 265–66.

What are some practical mechanisms we can employ toward that goal? When Steve Allison et al. (2003) surveyed literature on resilience they identified several prominent aspects of resilient functioning. These are presented above in table form, with examples of how the concepts may be used with providers. For our purposes, we are using CCSI Network Meetings where a family and multiple providers are present.

We have also found some useful tools in the resiliency work of psychologists Robert Brooks and Samuel Goldstein, whose writing and lectures have been very influential throughout our programs. In their book *The Power of Resilience* (2004) they posit ten ways in which individuals can nurture and develop resilient lifestyles, a development of thinking originally outlined by these same authors in *Raising Resilient Children* (2001). We have found several of these techniques applicable in helping shape systems of care to be more responsive organisms.

One such technique Brooks and Goldstein call "Making connections and displaying compassion" in which they stress the importance of remaining connected to others as a source of emotional well-being and resilience. The "charismatic adult," a person from whom we might gather strength, enhances this connection. Child development is, of course, immensely aided by the presence of a charismatic adult such as parent, teacher, therapist, or mentor. Group development and cohesive systems of care can similarly be influenced by an individual who will "step-up" and be a present advocate for a child—a risk-assumer—from whom the group can draw collective strength. This champion (who need not be a professional, as Saxe has pointed out) in a system of care will remind the group in subtle or not-so-subtle ways of its ability to "do better" and allow core strengths and hidden options to emerge and develop. As Brooks and Goldstein remind us, "even as adults we require charismatic adults in our lives" (2004, p. 16).

In the network group, where there are many adults, the charisma sometimes jumps like electricity from one member to another, and supplies everyone with renewed energy. Introductions always start off our meetings. We go around the room rattling off our names and titles. Once, after an adolescent introduced herself, the facilitator asked her age, then acknowledged how annoying adults could be—"We always ask your age and never share our own. I was asking so we would be sure not to offend you with suggestions that might be childish." The teen appreciated this explanation and gladly told her age, and added the additional information that her birthday was around Valentine's Day. The next person to introduce himself did so with name, occupation, and then added his age. Everyone laughed. The next provider introduced herself the same way, adding her advanced age with a heavy sigh. The group kept this up all the way around the table, adding interesting comments about their birth dates with the result that this network began with an intimacy and bonhomie that maintained itself for the duration of the meeting. Each member revealed their own brand of charisma and there were more cross-connections and gains made at this meeting than many others without such charismatic sharing.

The second set of techniques that help build resilient collaborations can be found under the mantle of "communicating effectively." Clinicians will be familiar with "active listening" where one attempts to understand and validate what other people are communicating as an effective therapeutic tool. Madsen (2007c) advocates collaboration as a process of "coresearch," or, "a partnership that taps the resourcefulness of clients and helpers" (p. 162). In work with clients "the process of eliciting, elaborating and acknowledging client abilities, skills and know-how can be powerfully transformative," according to Madsen, and we have found it to be similarly effective with groups representing systems of care. CCSI actively models this process in situ with children who are always included as a part of the planning group.

The technique of interviewing the child in the meeting affords participants an experience, rather than a report, of the person they may be entering into a partnership with. It's a conversation designed to reveal the child's charm, tenderness, humor, courage, or whatever engaging qualities they may possess. It is the centerpiece of the meeting and almost always elicits individual sparks of connection around the table. One provider after another spontaneously responds to something the child did, said, or alluded to, drawing them into new potential relationships.

In one such meeting a 16-year-old girl, sullen and nonverbal, seemed sure that this meeting was going to be just like every other she had been dragged to in the past. Her grandmother, sharing these doubts, was understandably protective and doing most of the talking. When the grandmother mentioned the girl's mechanical ability and how she liked to fix and build things, the facilitator capitalized on the moment. A toolbox full of new gear was lifted from under the table and plunked down in front of the teen. "I remember you told me," the facilitator said, "that you borrowed tools to make those wonderful bird houses I saw in your front yard. We thought you'd like your own starter box. Open it up and see." The teen's face transformed from bored, to disbelieving, then to sheer joy as she opened the box and removed tool after tool. She began to tell everyone what each implement was and how she intended to use it. From that moment on she was the "charismatic presence" that engaged the previously quiet group and initiated a variety of effective interactions with them.

Another time, a child with mild developmental delays, referred because of school refusal, sat shyly at the network table. He didn't feel competent to have a dialogue with this room full of professionals. The facilitator knew this boy, large for his age, was a prolific artist and could be gentle and sweet, though she had been warned prior to the home visit that he was physical, dangerous, and resistant. When it was clear he could not benefit from verbal discourse at the network meeting, the facilitator passed him paper and markers and asked if he could show what was keeping him from coming to school. He quickly drew and numbered three images: a chair, stairs, and a tiny blackboard. When he agreed that the participants could see his drawings the group responded with delight and genuine recognition of his skill. Because of their response he eagerly explained that (1) he did not fit in the tiny classroom chairs, (2) he became winded climbing the stairs, and (3) he could not see the blackboard from his seat in the rear of his classroom. He liked his teachers, classmates, and learning, but these practical barriers had been causing him great embarrassment. Because the meeting was not another shaming experience related to school, but instead a validating one where he could display a talent, a new level of communication was achieved that led to a quick resolution of a long-standing problem. His seat was replaced with an adult chair and moved to the front of the classroom. An agreement was formed whereby he could use the elevator while he participated in an exercise program to build muscles, reduce his weight, and help control his asthma.

Another aspect of communicating effectively is to control language, again through modeling, example, and at times active intervention from the facilitator. For example, at a case planning meeting in the clinic the family in question was being routinely referred to by role in a depersonalizing way: "mother said," "step-father complained," "brother did," and so on. A simple request to use proper names immediately had an impact on the discussion, reducing distance from the family. In the clinic we have learned that including the child and family in the room during systems-of-care discussions is the most powerful way of maintaining respectful communication patterns that in turn shape clinical thinking. Madsen has even devised a "client voice" exercise for when it is not possible to have actual clients in attendance. A clinician or group member is tasked with assuming the role of client and intermittently responding to the group "as if" they are the family member, thus deepening the group's empathic functioning.

It's easier to fall into deficit-based language when the client is not present. Even in medical procedures technicians use more decorum with a conscious patient than with those who are sedated. This is one reason the child is always present in their network meeting. Even so, there are times providers may slip into outdated or old habits. The facilitator must immediately respond to reframe such language. For example, a school psychologist turned to a child and said at a recent meeting, "You have to do 'X.'" The child responded by pulling back in her chair, and before any retort was uttered, the facilitator said, "She actually doesn't 'have' to do anything. Why do you think that course of action might be useful to her?" This took the focus off the child, defused what seemed to be a familiar argument, and reminded the provider of the task of this group.

At times it happens that the child in the meeting is quite comfortable addressing the adults with assertiveness and courage. Ironically, this can be more challenging to providers who may find they are feeling more defensive. In one such meeting a well-spoken, intelligent 16-year-old boy with a violent past and long history of institutionalization asked his psychiatrist why he could not go off the last bit of his medication, since everyone was reporting on how well he was doing. The psychiatrist replied that "they"—the team—were wary of negative behaviors and since they didn't find them yet, they wanted to wait a little longer. The CCSI coordinator, a guest at this meeting, listened to the ensuing pause for a moment, then turned to the psychiatrist and said, "You weren't really looking for negative behaviors, were you? You were looking for the therapeutic effect of your prescribed treatment, and you found it. It must be rewarding to have your treatment work so well. It's impressive, really, to hear how well Joe has been responding over this past year." The psychiatrist, a well-meaning clinician, responded to the recognition of his interventions and said, "Yes, it is rewarding. I'll look into halving the dose and see how well he does."

The strengths-based approach is not a set of techniques to be applied to consumers to reap better results. It is a way of believing about people—the ones we work with, and the ones we serve. When we turn our compassion onto fellow providers in the community it is because we can identify with their frustrations and barriers, and we trust that they have gifts to offer whether or not they are always demonstrated. People we serve live in complex communities. If the service providers do not know about one another they cannot work together, and if they do not have a model for working together valuable relationships go untried. We have found in our practice the most effective format for meetings of providers and families is one that utilizes aspects of strengths-based work with individuals. These focus on resilience, communicating respectfully, controlling language, and include the presence of charismatic others. Thus we do not relegate such an approach to individual work. We see it as the catalyst that effectively brings service systems to the table with children and families to give us all our best shot at influencing change.

## REFERENCES

Allison, S., Stacey, K., Dadds, V., Roeger, L., Wood, A., & Martin, G. (2003). What the family brings: Gathering evidence for strengths-based work. *Journal of Family Therapy, 25*, 263–284.

Brooks, R., & Goldstein, S. (2001). *Raising resilient children*. New York: McGraw-Hill.

Brooks, R., & Goldstein, S. (2004). *The power of resilience*. New York: McGraw-Hill.

Campbell, J. (1998). *Consumerism, outcomes and satisfaction: A review of the literature*. St. Louis, MO: Missouri Institute of Mental Health.

Don, M. (1997). *The sensuous garden*. New York: Simon & Schuster.

Greene, R. W., & Ablon, J. S. (2005). *Treating explosive kids: The collaborative problem-solving approach*. New York: Guilford.

Madsen, W. (2007a). *Collaborative therapy with multi-stressed families*. New York: Guilford Press.

Madsen, W. (2007b). "Sustaining collaborative practice in the 'real' world." Workshop Presentation Handout (pp. 1–18).

Madsen, W. (2007c). Working within traditional structures to support a collaborative clinical practice. *The International Journal of Narrative Therapy and Community Work, 2*, 51–61.

Morris, C. (1997). Mental health matters: Toward a non-medicalized approach to psychotherapy with women. *Women & Therapy, 20*(3), 63–77.

Norcross, J. (2002). *Psychotherapy relationships that work*. New York: Oxford University Press.

Rutter, M. (1999). Resilience concepts and findings: Implications for family therapy. *Journal of Family Therapy, 21*, 119–144.

Saxe, G., Ellis, H., & Kaplow, J. (2007). *Collaborative treatment of traumatized children and teens: The trauma systems therapy approach*. New York: Guiford.

Weiss, J. (1988). Substance versus symbol in administrative reform: The case of human services coordination. In C. Milofsky (Ed.), *Community organizations: Studies in resource mobilization and change* (pp. 100–135). New York: Oxford University Press.

# 16

# Strengths-Based Healing with Youth in Juvenile Detention

*John Soracco*

> Among all of the policy areas affecting vulnerable children and families, juvenile justice has probably suffered the most glaring gaps between best practice and common practice, between what we know and what we must often do. Perhaps because it serves an unpopular and powerless segment of our society—behaviorally troubled, primarily poor, mostly minority teenagers—juvenile justice policy has been too long shaped by misinformation, hyperbole, and political prejudices.
>
> —Annie E. Casey Foundation (2008, p. 1)

It was early on in my many years of experience working in the prison/detention system that I realized the hope that was present in juvenile detention settings was not necessarily a part of the adult corrections system. My frustrations occurred when I dealt with adult inmates who were incarcerated on many different occasions for the same type of criminal activity. In fact, I learned a true meaning of the phrase, "some people live and learn, and others just live."

A very rewarding time in my career, however, was when I ran a 60-bed facility for youthful offenders. In addition to my correction staff, I was permitted to have six adult offenders to serve as paraprofessionals. These men were selected from several prisons throughout the state. They were incarcerated for diverse offenses ranging from theft to murder. They were carefully screened by several layers of bureaucracy before they were approved to work in my program. The program divided 60 youth into 6 groups of 10, and each group was assigned a paraprofessional to run daily groups and address any situations as they occurred. My staff worked eight hours a day, five days a week and took off for vacations, holidays, and so on. The paraprofessionals were on the clock 24 hours a day, 7 days a week, with no time off. Their incentive was doing something rewarding with their time, and they would be provided with a good report to the state parole board.

The paraprofessionals were chosen from over 2,000 inmates throughout the adult system and considered it a privilege to work in my program for $1.24 per day. Several of the paraprofessionals were parents of teenagers; in fact, one of them had three teenage sons. I consider the program a tremendous success and the inmates that worked for me benefited greatly because they were respected for their strengths, which included leadership, compassion, and a desire to guide youth to help them avoid the path they might be headed on, toward long-term incarceration. The youth benefited in that they had positive role models that were with them every day, all day. I benefited in that I had mature leaders to supplement my staff.

I can best describe the strategies that in my experience worked best with juvenile youth by providing the following examples.

A youth came into the program who was trying to make a name for himself. He defied staff, refused to do schoolwork, and criticized every meal he was served. One day, the cook took this youth into the kitchen to separate him from others who he was negatively influencing. The cook had this youth help him prepare the dinner. This young man used the opportunity to creatively contribute toward the preparation of the food. When the meal was served, he was able to take pride and boasted how good it was going to be. This one simple strategy effectively changed the influence of this youth over the others from negative to positive.

Another time I worked in a community-based program. When youth acted out, it sometimes warranted calling the local police. Being a small rural community, many of the police were young and just starting a career in law enforcement. The youth were predominantly from larger cities and presented a challenge to these country police officers. Sometimes the attitude of the police incited the youth rather than calming them. After a conversation with the chief of police, it was decided that when a youth acted out, they would be assigned community service for their infraction. One of the community service chores would be to wash a patrol car. The stipulation was that the officer who brought the car would stay with the youth while the car was being cleaned. This most often resulted in a dialogue between the youth and the police officer. If the youth committed a new infraction, they had already somewhat of a rapport established, and their attitudes toward each other were much improved.

In my experience working with juveniles, I saw a definite hope for positive change as an individual grew, learned, and matured. At the end of this chapter, I share the story about the individual who confirmed in my mind that I would spend the rest of my career working with juvenile offenders.

Juvenile offenders who end up in locked detention centers suffer some of the worst outcomes of any youth cohort in our country. They are apt to achieve less educationally, work less and for lower pay, experience more family disruption, experience more chronic health problems, addiction, and more imprisonment (Chung, Little, & Steinberg, 2005). Long-term confinement does not seem to be the solution to dealing with our youth. Nor does confinement in large facilities where youth tend to get lost in the system while they learn more negative behaviors from their peers.

The adult system is one that punishes offenders for the crime they commit. Unfortunately, this same model is applied to institutions for youthful offenders. It should be understood that youth are inherently different from adults. Youth are, as a rule, more open to learning and more receptive to rehabilitation.

Children and adolescents, researchers clarified, are not just smaller versions of adults. New brain imaging research revealed that "the brain systems that govern impulse control, planning, and thinking ahead are still developing well beyond age 18" (Annie E. Casey Foundation, 2008, p. 6). It is well-established by research studies that adolescents remain far less able to gauge risks and consequences, control impulses, handle stress, and resist peer pressure. "Finally, research revealed that perhaps the most important difference between adolescent and adult lawbreakers is that most youthful offenders will cease lawbreaking as part of the normal maturation process" (Elliott, 1994, p. 18).

There have been cases where, due to the heinous nature of the crime, children as young as eight years old were presented to be treated as adults in the eyes of the court. Although I realize that these children cannot simply be returned to their home setting, locking them in a juvenile facility until they are 18, then transferring them to an adult facility is also not the answer. The many mitigating factors that cause this behavior have to be explored before an "individualized" treatment plan can be devised. We don't condone violence in any way, and everyone has to be accountable for their actions. If our understanding of the problem takes into account the complexities of causation, we will be able to be more effective in our efforts to prevent such tragedies.

In several documented cases, transferring youth to the adult criminal system resulted in more negative and more violent behaviors in later life. In order for a young person to transition from adolescence to adulthood, he or she must acquire marketable skills and education, as well as a social network. He must develop a sense of self-discipline and become independent. Incarceration too often denies these opportunities for youth, leaving the client unable to meet these necessary challenges of life.

Correction, by definition, is to modify undesirable behaviors that society determines need to be changed. Corrections indicate a focus on areas that need to be remedied, reformed, revised, and amended. It is a focus on the weaknesses and deficits that clients possess. It is a deficit-based approach, that doesn't focus on identifying potential strengths an individual might possess. In order for youth to grow and develop personal autonomy, they must be confident that they can achieve the task facing them. We talk about a comfort level, a personal space where we feel safe and confident. This comfort zone should include and even emphasize personal strengths, the talents we possess, are proud of, and that enhance our confidence. If asked, "what are the strengths you possess?" we could probably identify a few areas/talents. If we ask a youth in detention the same question, he or she would have a more difficult time with an answer. We often need to help youth identify their strengths. Over the years, I have employed several mechanisms to help youth identify their strengths. Some of the mechanisms I used include, but are not limited to, "Adventure Based Counseling" and "Circle of Courage."

## ADVENTURE BASED COUNSELING ACTIVITIES

Adventure Based Counseling is a therapeutic modality using experiential techniques to produce a lasting emotional and behavioral change in participants. These experiences are highly structured and sequenced to match the readiness of participants who are led through a series of activities designed to provide an increasing level of physical and emotional challenge.

The first activities are called *icebreakers* and concentrate on building group cohesion and improving individual comfort levels. These casual activities help the group to become more familiar with each other. The next level of participation includes activities designed to *decrease inhibitions*. They provide a slight increase in physical and emotional risk, while increasing the individual's commitment to the group. At this point, making a good effort is more important than success or failure at a particular task. The next series of activities are designed to develop *trust and empathy*. These activities ask each individual to trust his physical and emotional safety to others by attempting a graduated series of activities which involve taking some physical and/or emotional risks.

The next level of activities focuses on *communication*. In order to complete the physical activity, group members must share ideas and discuss possible solutions. During the activities, individuals with leadership abilities and skills usually emerge as group leaders. Once communication skills have evolved, *decision making and problem solving* exercises follow. Here, physical activity and verbal communication are involved in order to solve problems in activities that demand that group members demonstrate an ability to listen, cooperate, and compromise.

The sixth level of activities centers on *social responsibility*. Group success is somewhat dependent on each participant's ability to support and encourage the efforts of other participants. In these activities, youth are helped to learn the value of thinking and planning ahead rather than reacting in an impulsive and random manner, and there is a conscious effort on the part of facilitators to use metaphors to relate the group activity to the world "outside" in an empathetic and concerned manner.

Last in the series are the *personal responsibility* activities that are designed to help members acknowledge individual and common reactions to fear, stress, and physical limitation. These activities help young people extend the limits of their self-perceived competence and build self-confidence by successful completion of a difficult activity. Group members are helped to act on what they have learned about working cooperatively, supporting each other, and taking responsibility for one another's safety.

The sequenced activities draw out a variety of strengths in the youth. Many with physical capabilities excel in those activities requiring personal agility and strength. Those activities requiring communication, decision making, and problem solving allow for those with strengths in cognitive areas to excel. The teamwork required for these initiatives enable participants to identify and show pride in their areas of strength. As the activities progress, members of the team look to each other to help achieve personal, as well as group, goals. I have witnessed many teens gain new confidence in themselves and a better realization of what they can do well. We use these identified strengths in future counseling sessions while working with these youth. Adventure Based Counseling activities are based on the teachings of Project Adventure, Inc., of Hamilton, Massachusetts (see Schoel, Prouty, & Radcliffe, 1989).

## CIRCLE OF COURAGE

> They had what the world has lost. They have it now. . . . Be it for now or a hundred years from now, or a thousand—so long as the race of humanity shall survive—the Indian keeps his gift for us all.
>
> —John Collier (1947, p. 7)

Another method of strengths-based identification of natural gifts and talents which I have found to be helpful when working with youth can be found in the Circle of Courage model (Brendtro, Brokenleg, & Van Brockern, 1992). Traditional Native American child-rearing philosophies have provided us with unique perspectives of youth development. This child-rearing philosophy specific to the Lakota, or better known as the Sioux Native American People, focuses on identifying what gifts/strengths each individual possesses and how these gifts are used to interact with the world around them. The Lakota believe each person is born with natural gifts, strengths, and tendencies. It is when they realize their areas of strength that they can become most effective and valuable to themselves, as well as complementing different strengths in others.

Development of self-esteem is of primary importance in the socialization process of our youth. We have found this especially true in adolescents at risk, as their self-esteem tends to be underdeveloped due to a lack of a support system in their environment. The Lakota People, in developing the Circle of Courage, have identified four major areas of personal strengths and ways of interacting with others. Each area is commonly identified with a totem animal that expresses the characteristics of that spirit. These areas include mastery (buffalo), independence (eagle), generosity (deer), and belonging (bear). The exercise begins with an identification of each individual's gifts, as they see them, and a subsequent identification with a particular inclination. When participants are asked to identify their strength areas, they are provided with a gift identification listing or grid, which divides gifts into four categories (see grid below).

The first category would be those who see their strengths as being very goal-directed, quick to take action, like to be in control, and can generally be counted upon to get the job done. These people are referred to as buffaloes. They are the ones who put aside personal feelings and feelings of the group and concentrate at the task at hand. Their strengths lie in their abilities to complete any task in a timely and efficient manner.

The next area of gift identification would be those persons who possess great vision, who have an eye toward the future. They are generally creative and imaginative. They are the ones who see the big picture. Their strengths lie in their ability to visualize a need to plan for the future as well as the creative ideas to attain that goal. These people are referred to as eagles, and they are idea people.

The next category of gift identification would include characteristics of those who are supporting, trusting, and caring. They are the people who value harmony and social cohesiveness. They possess great people-skills. They tend to be charismatic and find satisfaction in helping others. These people are associated with the deer. Their affinity for harmony is most important in their dealings in life.

The next area of gift identification would include those who are known as the keepers of tradition. They are the people who pay attention to detail, need to have and follow rules and procedures, and are practical in their dealings with others. They tend to be analytical. These people are associated with the bear. They are information gatherers and need to have all the data before making decisions.

## IDENTIFY YOUR GIFTS

Examine the four boxes below and choose the one that *best* describes your gifts.

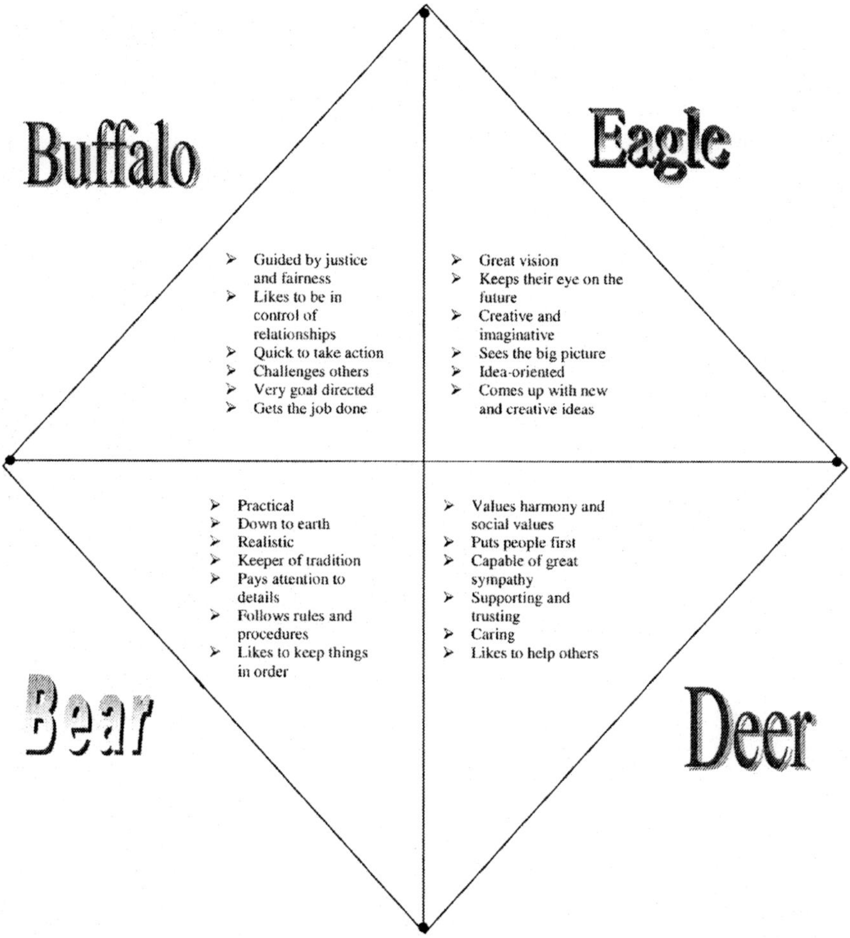


**Figure 16.1. Four Areas of Personal Strength**

Once a person identifies his gifts or area of strengths, he will better understand how he or she can be of value to the group as well as understand the dynamics of what drives people who identify with other groups. Once a person has this understanding, he or she can adapt or flex to meet other people's styles. In addition to possessing gifts, this exercise also points out that inherent in some gift categories are limitations. For example, buffalo people can tend to be autocratic. They can trample their way through a project and not realize the stress they may be causing others. Conversely, the deer people might be unfairly taken advantage of because they place so much value on harmony that they cannot say no, when sometimes they should. Eagle people can tend to have their heads in the clouds and come up with ideas that may not be feasible or logical. Bear people can become mired in the details and may get little "real" work done if not prodded.

Once the strength and limitations of these personality categories are understood and accepted, a holistic team can be formed. All styles are necessary to make a group complete. The four styles complement each other in achieving this wholeness. When presenting this modality to youth, the understanding of the four styles is as important as identifying personal strengths and gifts. When an individual is a part of a group and he or she is appreciated and praised for his or her input, he or she is generally willing to take more emotional risks. Youth are taught that they will receive praise for using their gifts to further the group cause but are also constantly reminded that they must be tolerant of other people's gifts and limitations. The buffalo seldom has time for the compassion of the deer. The eagle wants to create and not be accountable to the bear for statistics to support all his or her ideas. The Lakota teach us that all people are born with gifts and we should look for these strengths in people if we are to benefit from their input. The motto is "None of us is as smart as all of us!"

## CASE STUDY I: "WHY I CHOSE JUVENILE, RATHER THAN ADULT, CORRECTIONS: LIFE ON THE INSTALLMENT PLAN"

Many years ago, when I was working in adult corrections piloting a new community-based/halfway-house program, I worked with Mike. The goal of the program was to transition inmates from the adult prison system back into the community. The tasks of the program were to help the inmates attain employment, further their education, and solidify family bonds, among others. The inmates that were chosen for the program were those who showed potential while in the adult system and an ability to function in a supervised community program. Since employment was viewed as a key factor in success, enabling inmates to achieve independence through an ability to become self-supporting was heavily emphasized.

When Mike entered the program, he had family ties that enabled him to achieve employment during his first week in the program. The job was driving a fuel truck that delivered home heating oil. He reported to work on time, he seemed happy with his employer, his wage was significantly higher then many of the other working inmates, and he was well on his way to successful adjustment into the program.

One evening, while I was working late, I had a visit from a sergeant and a patrol officer from a local police department. They asked me if Mike was part of the program, if he was employed, where he was employed, and what he did for the company. I supplied the information that they requested but asked why they were doing this investigation. They replied that this particular company was under suspicion of removing fuel oil from customers' tanks without the customers' knowledge and that they were going to set up a sting for the following day.

When Mike came in that night, I questioned him about how his job was going and exactly what his function was for the company. He responded that even though he drove a delivery truck, his job was to remove oil from people's tanks. I asked why he would be removing oil, and he stated that he guessed that there was something wrong with the oil, or that the tank needed cleaning, or that there was a possible leak, and gave me several more reasons for removing oil. At that point, he became suspicious of my questioning and asked why I was so interested in his job. I then asked if he ever spoke with any of the people whose tanks he was emptying as to why oil was being removed. He replied, "No," and became even more suspicious and stated to me that if I thought he was stealing from people, that I was dead wrong. But he also realized that something was amiss.

At that point, he insisted I go get his jacket (file). I asked him why, since I knew why he had been incarcerated since age 13. He said he needed to show me something. When I brought his folder to the office, it reflected that his criminal history began at an early age, and every charge in his record had to do with physical violence. He had charges for assault and battery, assault with intent, assault with a deadly weapon . . . any charge that the word assault could be associated with seemed to be present on this record. I asked what point he was trying to make, and he stated, "Do you see any theft charges at all?" I replied, "No." And his comment was, "I never stole anything from anybody" and he wasn't about to start now. Mike truly believed that this was an admirable quality and a true strength that he possessed.

I believed that he was unaware of any wrongdoing, and I demanded that he not go to work the next day. His reply was that he was going to go out and "get them" for setting him up. I replied that he wasn't "getting anybody for anything" since he would not be leaving the house. He then complied with my directive. The next day, the sting went down, the company was held accountable, and arrests were made. Later that day, Mike came into my office, thanked me for saving him from going back to prison for something that he still insisted he had no part or knowledge of, and stated that he owes me one and, "if I ever need anyone taken care of, just to let him know." That's when I coined the phrase, "Life on the installment plan," knowing well that Mike would not be going to jail for theft, but there were high odds of him going back for crimes of a physical nature. This man truly believed that his strength was in the fact that he was not a thief. He gave no second thoughts to the fact that other crimes of a physical nature were okay with him.

On the other hand, once I was dealing with a youth who stole his parents' car and went joyriding. When he came to detention and we were discussing what he did, I asked, "What were you thinking?" and with a very innocent look, he responded, "Oh, I wasn't thinking." There is a big difference between an adult that has decided what is right and wrong for himself, versus a youth who is not mature enough to make good, socially responsible decisions.

The differences in the ethical thought process and rationalization between youth and adults convinced me that I preferred working with juveniles versus adults.

## CASE STUDY II: ADVENTURE BASED COUNSELING—WHEN JAMES REALIZED THAT HE WASN'T ALWAYS EXPECTED TO HAVE THE BEST SOLUTION TO ALL THE PROBLEMS

On a bright, crisp September morning, a group of youth was escorted to a field still wet with the morning dew. As expected, they were excited about the pending adventure, but all became involved in the contagious complaining about why they had to start so early . . . the grass was wet . . . expensive sneakers were being ruined. . . . As a matter of practice, I ignored the complaints as I retorted with positive comments about the weather and the fun we were about to have. The common practice when using the Adventure Based Counseling course was to have the house manager, in this case James, and his assistant manager accompany their group. On this particular morning, two youth had gotten into a fight (undoubtedly in an attempt to show their strengths) and James and his assistant were not able to start the day with their group. Experience taught me to start the activities as planned, because waiting provided idle time, which was not a productive way to start a day. The activities began.

Since the group had done several activities on a previous occasion, we progressed directly to those initiatives involving decision making and problem solving. The young people completed two activities, and then we processed the events. The entire group participated and contributed to the decisions of the group as to how to achieve their goals. We were about finished with a second set of activities when James and his assistant arrived. They sat out on the activity, as it had already begun.

When we gathered to process, the youth were quiet. None of the youth contributed, but instead looked to James for leadership. The manager gave his assessment and presented his ideas, which were all accepted by the youth. As the facilitator, I observed that prior to the arrival of the managers the youth viewed processing as their responsibility. However, they gave up this responsibility to a person of authority. The irony was that the youth actually came up with better assessments and ideas than the managers. We continued the processing, and I asked the managers to sit quietly and allow the youth to lead the discussion. Some youth were a bit intimidated by this request, but others had no problem participating in this exercise. James and his assistant complied and were amazed at the contributions that the youth were capable of making. This eventually changed a "top-down" attitude to one of placing value upon the insight, input, and strengths of the youth, allowing for greater acceptance of youth ideas in the future. The teens also greatly benefited as their input was valued, and this encouraged them to want to actively participate in discussions that affected their future.

## CASE STUDY III: CIRCLE OF COURAGE— RICARDO USED THE LESSON TO JUDGE OTHERS

The goal of the Circle of Courage exercise is to help people identify their own strengths and the limitations which are inherent with any gifts. I once was asked to present the Circle of Courage exercise to a group of teenagers who were participating in a federally funded summer employment program. As we proceeded through the exercise, the youth all seemed to benefit from the initiative. The interaction was great. The comment, "Now I know why you act like you do" echoed throughout the room. When we discussed how we would use our strengths for the upcoming employment, Ricardo commented that he knew who he was, but would use this lesson to figure out others. When asked what he meant, he relayed a story about how he lost three previous jobs because he didn't figure his boss out until it was too late. He told the group that one of his bosses was a "buffalo" and if he knew how those personalities were, he would have moved faster and completed the task quicker. In another job, Ricardo had a "deer" for a boss, and he took advantage of this kindness. He would come to work late, take long breaks, and often asked to leave early. As nice as his boss was, the decision was to let Ricardo go, he was fired.

Ricardo said that as a result of this exercise, now he would figure out what personality traits his bosses have and make sure that he acted accordingly. Ricardo kept the job for the duration of the summer program—a true achievement!

## SUMMARY

The youth I have worked with throughout my career are mostly inner-city youth who have been exposed to extremely stressful and pathological environments, combined often with a harsh and dysfunctional family atmosphere and poverty. Despite these heavy weights, the will to survive and thrive was strong.

I have always found that it is more rewarding to give than to receive. During the holiday season, many groups want to give gifts, cookies . . . to our youth. The kids are generally on the receiving end, and it seems that the more they get, the more they expect. We reversed this by having the youth prepare a meal for the local fire department every September 11th. The youth prepare and serve the meal, then provide an audience for those firefighters to tell their stories of September 11, 2001. You can see in the faces of the youth that the appreciation they are shown for their effort is truly rewarding.

We all have strengths/gifts. It's when we are able to identify and put these strengths to work that we achieve. Simply put, if we like what we are doing because we are confident in ourselves, we will most likely do a better job. This confidence comes from doing what we do best—exercising our strengths.

## REFERENCES

Annie E. Casey Foundation. (2008). *A road map for juvenile justice reform*. Baltimore, MD.

Brendtro, L., Brokenleg, M., & Van Bockern, S. (1992). *Reclaiming youth at risk—our hope for the future*. Bloomington, IN: National Educational Service.

Brief of the American Medical Association et al., as Amici Curiae in Support of Respondent, *Roper v. Simmons*, 543 U.S. 551 (2005) (No. 03-633), available at www.abanet.org/crimjust/juvjus/simmons/ama.pdf.

Chung, H. L., Little, M., & Steinberg, L. (2005). The transition to adulthood for adolescents in the juvenile justice system: A developmental perspective. In D. W. Osgood, E. M. Foster, C. Flanagan, & G. R. Ruth (Eds.), *On your own without a net: The transition to adulthood for vulnerable populations* (pp. 68–91). Chicago: University of Chicago Press.

Collier, J. (1947). *The Indians of the Americas*. New York: W. W. Norton.

Elliott, D. S. (1994). Youth violence: An overview. Paper presented at The Aspen Institute's Children's Policy Forum, Children and Violence Conference. Queenstown, MD.

Schoel, J., Prouty, D., & Radcliffe, P. (1989). *Islands of healing: A guide to adventure based counseling*. Hamilton, MA: Adventure Based Counseling.

# 17

# A Home of Healing and Reverence

*Renee Fillette*

Our work with children is nothing less than a relentless pursuit to find the most direct path to their souls and whisper a lingering mantra: "You are filled with amazing potential beyond my dreams for you. You are beautiful [and perfect] just as you are. You are wanted. You are needed. You have a purpose."

## HOW WE UNDERSTAND THESE VULNERABLE YOUTH

### A Friendly Abduction

I sometimes wonder if, through the child's experience, their removal from their home feels like a friendly abduction into the Land of Oz, with winding roads, new friends and foes around each corner, and their deepest longings encapsulated in the words, "There's no place like home." Armed with best intentions, and clinical expertise, we, child care professionals, persevere in caring for these tender souls as they make their way in a foreign land on a quest to find home. With this privilege of guiding youth to places yet unknown, we have the responsibility of constant self-evaluation and self-reflection, certain that we always lead with compassion, virtue, and respect.

In an effort to restore the vitality that has been lost through traumatic childhood experiences, and mend the gaping wounds of disrupted relationships and lost connections, we offer children a home for healing. Usually a child arrives at our front door after they have been displaced from multiple foster families, or have resided in an institutional environment for some time and are ready to live in the community. Each group home is occupied by no more than six youth who are cared for by a team of counselors, a house parent, and a social worker. The homes are all located within a community setting where the children live unsheltered from the world around them. In many ways the organization is run from the bottom up, with those who spend the most time caring for our youth having a loud voice in program development. The children themselves are regularly empowered to contribute to how their home and life is managed with open access to all levels throughout the organization. We are in a constant state of development, learning from one another and supporting each other to grow.

## Empty Spaces

For most of our youth, the absence of a parent in their lives creates an empty cavern, impossible to fill, leaving behind a hurt that is without consolation. The stories of Ben and Emma articulate a common thread in our experiences caring for youth, and reveal the profound resilience that has breathed life into each of us who has touched their pain. They exemplify the power of fortitude, need for family, and fierce resolve that, if viewed from a strengths-based perspective, can be considered their greatest gifts.

### *Ben*

Ben moved into our home when he was 11. His mother used drugs throughout her pregnancy and continued through much of his turbulent life. Shortly after his birth, his parents separated and Ben was shuffled between friends and family members, never staying in one place for more than a few months. Upheaval, displacement, and chaos became the familiar ebb and flow of his early years. It was not uncommon for him to spend weekdays in one house and weekends in another. His early childhood was characterized by constant disruption, violence, exposure to drug abuse, and his mother's schizophrenic episodes. Throughout his formative years Ben was physically and sexually abused, and shuffled between hospitals, group homes, and several foster families.

Ben learned to adapt to each new environment by taking control and eliciting the disruptions before someone else made the decision to reject him again. As he began to feel comforted by the stability of a new placement, his emotional armor surfaced and he would break windows, punch holes in walls, or assault his caregiver. He often paced, groaned, cried, and tugged at himself in an effort to soothe away the pain. Over time his aggression was more often directed toward his mother and later whoever played a maternal role. Unable to fathom a stable living environment, Ben watched from a distance as his two younger half-siblings enjoyed the affections he was unable to access from grandparents and extended family. He had burned bridges with his family and foster families such that no doors were left open to him. His early life experiences had created caverns of despair from where emerged a child no one felt they could manage for more than a few days. Eventually both of Ben's parents forbade him from contacting them. As a final effort to keep him from residential placement, Ben was referred to our group home.

Within the first few months of settling into our family-style home, Ben thrived. He was able to reveal his capacity to learn and grow in a new school, and to forge deep bonds with his five housemates. Surprisingly, a solid foundation was easily set and attachments were strengthening. We often found ourselves perplexed as to why so many people in his life had rejected him, leaving him so alone. It wasn't until six months into his placement at our home that Ben showed signs of emotional distress and behavioral regression. Weeks before each holiday he was in a state of heightened agitation. His innate need for his family became compulsive as he rang for his mother over and over, blocking the number each time, hoping she might answer if she didn't identify his number calling. His calls would go out to aunts, former foster families, family friends, and grandparents, always with a plea to come home. Each unanswered call tore away the recent scabs from his healing wounds. Following each round of unsuccessful calls were bouts of anger and destruction, ending with the sobbing lament, "I just want my mom. I promise I can be better."

Our work, our mantra whispered to his soul, was intended to somehow ground him long enough for him to be able to take stock of his situation and settle within our home. By identifying his strengths as his unrelenting resilience, his humor, and his intellect, the team focused on building his sense of self-worth. Here is where the real work was done. First, Ben's deep, unquenchable need for his mother and family were recognized and honored. The team was actively empathic and sympathetic to his situation. Frequent opportunities were given for him to talk about and act out his pain. Ben was given the liberty of time alone in his fort, long walks, and calls to people who we knew would answer the phone. Ben needed someone to call, and the team became the ones who agreed to answer the phone. Everyone, from the executive director to off-duty child care counselors, agreed to answer Ben's calls day or night.

Next, an emphasis was placed on building Ben's capacity to have the same fun that his peers enjoyed. He played on a local baseball team, joined scouts, and met his friends at the movies on Friday nights. When his emotions interfered, the team coaxed him to rely on the relationships he had built with teachers and mentors, connections that evolved from his academic success. At those moments he would be given extra attention in school, used as a positive example to his peers, and asked to tutor other students. He would feel empowered by this success, and this translated to the ability to better regulate his emotions. The team also encouraged him to use his uncanny sense of humor to rally his friends around him, and provide him with the support he needed.

Most poignantly perhaps are the stories of contributions from the other boys in the house. Through them the home began to fill the bottomless cavern of Ben's emptiness, and affirm that he was an essential member of the group. As the cycle was triggered, Ben would inevitably act out in an attempt to foment a disruption in his placement. Tensions would rise. After pacing, and making fruitless calls to his family, Ben would try to burn himself, run away, or destroy parts of the house. Other times he would run to the local park and plead with strangers to take him away somewhere—anywhere. These episodes were separated with periods of peace and laughter, unexpectedly interrupted again with explosions of rage and despair. As the team and clinicians sought after the key to help Ben accept our commitment to care for him, without condition, it became clear that the boys themselves could move him to the place he feared most—a sense of belonging and stability. After a major eruption, the boys would sit together and speak from their hearts to Ben, letting him know how much he meant to them, and how the house wouldn't be the same if he wasn't there. They would ask him not to leave, and reassure him of his place among them. This practice became enriching not only to Ben, but to the other boys who found strength and empowerment in the power of their compassion for their housemate. Boys who had otherwise felt helpless and unneeded themselves so often, had found purpose in their camaraderie. They were not isolated entities existing beneath the same roof, rather young men with traumatic pasts who could derive strength from one another and forge a new life for themselves.

This progress could not happen, however, without the absolute commitment of everyone throughout the organization. As Ben attempted to undermine his placement, pulling out all of the strategies that had worked in the past, it became increasingly important for the staff throughout the agency to be consciously aware of the reasons he was behaving this way, and the negative consequences of giving in to his desire to be relocated for the sake of movement. When we recognized the burning desire to be reunited with his family at the core of Ben's struggle, we could find unflinching empathy and compassion for him. When we lost sight of this fundamental need our children have, we relinquished a part of our humanity. While at the surface the issue appeared to be a push and pull for chores to be done, use of the telephone, and privileges within the community, there was often a much more powerful force at work beneath the obvious. Open conversations with staff and Ben, training, and constant communication were essential in bringing these motives to the surface. Our work with children is without purpose if we resign ourselves to power struggles. Our presence in their lives is nothing less than toxic when we steal their voices and stop listening to their cry for help.

Through repetition, communication, and enduring commitment to keeping Ben grounded in his new home through each crisis, a new template for family living began to develop for him. A new point of reference began to emerge at long last so that when his anxiety, anger, and depression began to overwhelm him, rather than resorting to self-abuse and destruction in hope of disrupting his placement, he grabbed hold of what he identified as "family" and reached out for help. As these new behaviors replaced former ones, the word spread to Ben's family and an interest in spending time with him began to emerge. While these contacts were often accompanied by painful episodes of regression for Ben, his placement in his group home was never compromised and he was free to renegotiate his relationship with his family within the safety net our home.

*Emma*

Emma's emotional wounds were gaping and raw when she came to us. After years of fruitless searches for her mother, she couldn't stop running. Day and night, from home and school, Emma ran. Sometimes she would be gone for a few minutes, other times for days. She was a familiar face to local police, who had been called countless times to search for her. We negotiated deals with Emma to encourage her not to run, taped signs to the doors listing meaningful reasons not to leave, and pleaded with her to stay. Team meetings were occupied with answering the question, "Where was Emma going?" The answer remained, "To find her mother." Although her mother's incarceration separated them when she was three, Emma never lost hope of reuniting with her. The behaviors that grew from her unquenchable thirst could not be deterred with rewards or punishment. There was no convincing her to stop. Often her journeys lacked any direction or viable information as to where her mother might be; still she could not be dissuaded.

Not only did Emma run from the group home, but she ran from intimate connections with people who cared for her. Attachments had to be created through invisible attempts to connect with her. Otherwise, they were doomed. Emma cleverly sabotaged foster family placements and attempts to adopt her throughout the years, desperately holding tight to the fantasy of reunifying with her mother.

The work of grounding Emma seemed impossible for months upon months. Attempts to help her focus on accomplishments in school were in vain. Therapy sessions, individualized plans for helping her manage, giving her a private bedroom, even dedicating one special member of the team to work with her all failed to keep her from running. The team agreed to come to work with sneakers on and be prepared to run. Whenever possible we stayed right behind her, reminding her with our words and actions that we would not leave her. One of Emma's greatest strengths was her intense desire for lasting intimate connections with people, but because she could not find it in herself to trust people not to abandon her, she constructed an obstacle course of walls too high and ravines too deep for anyone to reach her. When Emma's running continued to place her in danger we grew concerned that we could no longer ensure her safety. We made the difficult decision to move her to a higher level of care where she could not easily run away.

The commitment to a child does not end with a negative discharge such as this. In fact, it is at this critical time that the relationship becomes even more important. With the team's understanding that once accessible, Emma's capacity for connecting with people would be a source of her resilience, the decision was made to make a special effort to maintain contact with her. Phone calls, letters, and visits maintained the connection during the time apart, whether Emma was planning to return to the group home or not. It was essential that Emma know and feel that the relationships that had been forged with members of the team were not going to be abandoned. Those relationships meant quite a lot, and they could be relied upon, especially in times of need. Emma could feel this, and the residents who remained in the group home now had an intimate understanding of the authenticity of the relationships they themselves had with the team. This trust could ease the tension and anxiety that framed so much of their experience in the foster care system.

After she left us, Emma's journey eventually included a brief stay with a foster family, a hospitalization, and a return to a residential treatment center. We never lost touch. When it came time for her to be discharged back to a lower level of care, our group home was the natural choice for her. Emma tapped into her strengths by advocating for her return to us. She composed heartfelt letters to her county case workers, family court judge, and to us. At the age of 16 she orchestrated her own discharge and ensured her return to our home.

While we welcomed Emma back to us with open arms, there was still an enormous amount of work to be done. Our contacts with her had only begun to scratch the surface of her potential for building strong, lasting attachments. Following a brief honeymoon period, her old dysfunctional coping mechanisms returned and the elopements began again. This time her adventures included drug use, refusing to go to school, and engaging in sexually promiscuous activities. Exhausted from the mere memory of sleepless nights worrying for her, the team took a strong approach. We reminded her, again, that we would not leave her. We reminded her of our commitment to her and of how it had endured through time and place. But, we would not allow her to place herself at risk again. The thought of leaving the group home again resonated within her deeply enough to effect change this time. Emma advocated for one final opportunity to make a change. Our requests of her were simple, it seemed to us. We asked that she not run away, not use drugs, and go to school every day. In exchange she could expect to return home each afternoon to a place of warmth and dependability. The low rate of turnover among staff (0 percent in over two years) meant that there was consistency in care and genuine concern for her. Emma could count on us to care for her unabashedly, with open doors and open hearts. She was able to hear our message, to trust in our words, and to agree to move forward with us. From that moment forward she attended school, stopped engaging in unsafe behaviors, and stopped running away.

Three months into the enjoyment of Emma's success the social workers called to say that Emma's mother had been released from prison and wanted to see her. The initial reaction of the team was to protect Emma, and themselves, from the disruption this would bring to a fragile, newly settled child. Holding our breath and fingers tightly crossed, we hoped that our strengths-based approach with Emma had provided her with the resources she needed to rely so heavily upon during the reintroduction to her mother.

Emma watched closely as our team quickly embraced her mother, without judgment, and welcomed her into our home. She was confident in following our lead and soon began exposing the raw, unhealed wounds that only this reunion could mend. She greeted her mother as an insightful, resilient, and securely attached adolescent. While the road remained bumpy for Emma, she faced each day at school regardless of the disruptions in her personal life, and continued to progress toward physical and emotional independence.

## OUR TREATMENT PHILOSOPHY

### The Enduring Connection

For so many vulnerable children, foster care is characterized by multiple placements, staff turnover, and artificial relationships that end abruptly when they are discharged. By focusing on relationships and shifting attention from rewards and punishments to intimate connections between youth and caregivers, strong bonds are forged that become a sustaining resource for support. It is our common practice not to abandon our children when they leave, but to remain a beacon of light to reference whenever needed. This has had positive implications beyond our expectations for our children, families, and staff.

The staff derives immeasurable gratification and validation when they have the opportunity to reconnect with a former resident. No matter the circumstance surrounding the contact, whether it be in times of triumph or times of trouble, the opportunity to offer continued support and water the soil where seeds had been planted is inspiring and contagious. With a structured format in place for maintaining ethical boundaries, communication between the discharged youth and former caregivers at the organization can endure. This means answering a call for help, going to visit, encouraging through tough times, celebrating successes, and listening. When current residents are exposed to the connection we maintain with youth who have been discharged, there is an understanding that they too will have a touchstone for when their journey takes them to distant places.

## Group Home Tenets

Our experience has been that children living away from their families need a sense of hope and purpose. This is a soulful and deeply individualized process in which the team needs to understand from where the child's sense of purpose originates. For some, the answer is obviously their desire to return home and to be the son or daughter and sibling they were intended to be. For others, the answer is elusive and significant time and energy needs to be focused on identifying that place. The process of achieving one's purpose is among four primary tenets that our group home team emulates in their daily work:

1. Understand that relationships can be relied upon, negotiated, and healed.

When a child comes to us he often leaves behind him a trail of ruptured relationships with parents, siblings, extended family, foster families, and friends who have attempted, unsuccessfully, to heal his wounds. At the group home, relationships are established under terms of reciprocal respect and understanding. The work begins with the child care counselor's ability to see beyond ferocious behaviors and timid withdrawals, into the hidden child who has only been temporarily transformed in response to his once-volatile environment. Renegotiating these new terms to the child-caregiver relationship requires patience, compassion, and remarkable endurance from both the child and the counselor. This evolving negotiation becomes the template for future, more intimate relationships.

2. We are, each of us, a work in progress.

Accepting that each of us is fallible, and developing patience and compassion for each other's mistakes, is an important life lesson that is emphasized in the group home. Keeping this mind-set in the forefront of our minds helps us to eliminate the dangerous pitfalls of creating an overly authoritative and controlling environment in our home. While clearly there is an understanding that the adults guide, direct, instruct, coach, and protect the youth, status does not imply flawless decision making. This realization can be a humbling experience; one that encourages communication and negotiation rather than a damaging struggle for power.

3. Everyone needs a sense of purpose and a means for accomplishing the goal.

When children have no viable family resource to return home to, it becomes critically important to help them understand that they do indeed have a purpose. For one youth whose parents both died while he lived in our group home, his sense of purpose was derived from helping the younger, disabled children in his school. He found his niche in caring for children who he interpreted to be more vulnerable than him, and found a source for his own strength and resilience in helping others. This work speaks specifically to a strengths-based ideology; it establishes a baseline for the capacity to be a contributing member to one's community, be it family, group home, or school, and builds on what already exists within the child.

4. Youth must be empowered to be who they are, not who we intend for them to be.

As caretakers of our youth we can become easily persuaded to guide them in the direction we see fit rather than opening the doors along the path of their choice. This requires making use of frequent opportunities to pause and reflect about the purpose of our work together and to constantly align ourselves with the individual goals of each child. If a child wants to become an illustrator when he grows up, it is our responsibility to find a way to help him make choices that will lead him there. If a child wants to live in an environment we consider to be less than optimal, it becomes our inherent responsibility to teach him the skills he will need to survive in that situation.

This notion is especially true when a youth seeks to reestablish or maintain relationships with family members who have mistreated or neglected them in the past. Regardless of a parent's rights being legally terminated, or a history of extreme abuse and neglect, very often youth hold on to the fantasy of a mended relationship with their family. We believe strongly that when adolescents express this, and feel committed to pursuing this relationship at all cost, it is often in their best interest to safely facilitate that connection. With assistance from therapists and clinically skilled child care counselors, this opportunity to navigate treacherous and uncertain waters is better done when the youth has a safe harbor to return to after the storm. If we deny this connection, we leave the adolescent to emancipate himself from the foster care system, and to attempt to understand the dynamics and emotions of complex and intimate relationships without a guide.

## Guidelines

The overarching goal at our group home is not to teach our youth how to navigate a system of rewards and punishments, rather to find meaning and purpose in making the best decision while considering the impact on others. To that end we have chosen not to employ a token or level system, or any other form of extrinsic reward system. We have decided together that maladaptive behaviors would be interpreted before they are reacted to, and an emphasis would be placed on building skills to overcome maladaptive behavior patterns rather than simply punishing them. By replacing disruptive behaviors with adaptive behaviors, and relying upon the intrinsic gratification of that new behavior, we begin to reshape individual behaviors and entire patterns of relationships.

It was our experience that there is a natural tendency for youth and adults to share a mutual understanding of a firm set of rules by which the house is structured. In the development of a set of rules for the houses, there was an urge to create a list of do's and don'ts that was directed toward the youth and their behavior. The team asked for a written list of expectations, with specific consequences for breaking each rule. If a child cursed, the team wanted a consequence. If the child broke the television set, a much bigger consequence. The premise behind this thinking is that the punishments would be proportional to fit the infraction, and deter the youth from similar choices in the future. Another assumption for this method of child rearing was that it would enable the team, who worked in shifts, to be absolutely consistent with each other's expectations. Some staff felt this would provide them with the leverage and authority they needed to control the environment and the children. I did not agree.

Our aim was never to control the children. While we recognize the importance of providing an environment that the youth can consistently count on, in the real world people are not absolutely consistent with each other and they do not follow a script when reacting to behaviors in a relationship. From the outset of the project we were intending to guide the youth, providing them with opportunities to make choices that were both good and bad, and to ease them into understanding and accepting the natural consequences of those choices. We were especially concerned not to create a relationship with teens that encouraged them to focus on learning how to navigate our system to maximize rewards and minimize punishments.

Our strategy was to offer the young people a home where they had freedom of choice in all areas, with natural consequences for those choices. A baseline set of expectations was established for which no tangible rewards were given. This meant that making one's bed, cleaning dishes, doing household chores that contribute to the shared living space, going to school, and treating others with respect was not rewarded with tokens, money, or any other tangible item. These behaviors are rudimentary for survival in any home, or relationship, and the motivation for successful participation in these activities is the intrinsic satisfaction that is derived from knowing you have made those around you happy. This philosophy of treatment, we believe, is a critical component of our work with the youth, and a method that encourages generalization to their caregivers and partners beyond the scope of their foster care placement.

Similarly, when a youth chooses not to keep up with the basics of daily living in the home, natural consequences will follow. For example, if a child disrupts a community outing by cursing and leaving the group, then it will be some time before that child will be invited to go on a group outing again. There is no arbitrarily selected time period for which the child is not allowed to go out with the group, rather an agreed upon expectation that the child will somehow demonstrate improved impulse control. There is no prescribed period of grounding, rather an understanding that the child acted this way because of a lack of ability in a certain skill area, and the team and child work together to build the capacity for success. Missing out on fun trips becomes a motivating factor for the youth to develop and demonstrate the skills required to go, and the lack of an ability to simply punish the child inspires the staff to work with the child to gain the skills rather than to passively wait at home and "control" the youth.

Negotiating relationships with our youth in this way is challenging for both the children and the staff. Caring for our children can be an emotionally daunting task, and it is natural to search for the path of least resistance. It's common to want to manage the immediate situation rather than invest time and energy forecasting into the future. In the midst of a volatile explosion of emotions, it is challenging for the child care counselor to ask oneself how best to handle the situation so that the adolescent learns from the interaction and carries the lesson with them. In some moments it can be nearly impossible to see the big picture. It's through constant communication, supervision, training, and peer support that child care counselors are better able to step back from the immediacy, and react with a set of tools that builds strengths and character. There is no place for intimidation, authoritative posturing, or bullying. The only gain is through patience and consistent skill building. When we have manipulated the environment to such an extent that youth have learned how to behave when it is to their advantage, but beneath the surface there is only an interest in personal gain, we have failed. When we impart new skills upon our youth that become intrinsically motivating, we till fertile soil where successful relationships can flourish with family members, friends, and partners, we have done good work.

## Our Families

An individual's need for a family connection can be a powerful force in building one's strengths and an opportunity for reconfiguring old patterns of familial dysfunction. Whether a child comes to us with a family of permanence, or not, the relationship between the child and their family remains at the core of our work. While there is remarkable variation in the types of relationships our youth may have with their families, from full parental involvement to severed communication, each child wrestles with understanding why and how it all came to be, and where to go from here. An empathic understanding of this sometimes painful situation is a shared responsibility of all of us within the organization.

In its early stages, the family-organization relationship is a fragile connection where parents and staff proceed cautiously down an uncertain path. In its finest form, parents are unified with child care staff, effectively coparenting the child, building the families' strengths and capacity until reunification is possible and long-term success is most eminent. As this essential relationship develops, we note three factors that significantly influence the core connection: trust, acceptance, and communication.

Our work to preserve and restore families requires constant and mutual authenticity. As administrators and child care staff, we are invested in an almost daily pursuit to earn a family's trust so that a genuine connection can be formed. While maintaining professional etiquette, we also reveal a very human and empathic face in our work. We ask that families trust that we have an understanding of their child and the unique complexities of their family dynamic enough for us to be able to offer value. We hope for the privilege of a glimpse into the very real challenges the families confront, so that we can best honor their circumstance and offer our help. For some, we find open doors, receptive to our intrusion and intervention. For others, we experience an initial resistance so profound that it can only be borne out of the trauma and intense volatility of the separation of parent from child—a disruption that cannot be easily reconciled. For these children and their families we offer a sometimes unwelcome hand, and an absolute commitment of honesty.

Without exception, we accept the bags and burdens of each family, without judgment. Our focus is to understand and respect the familial culture, the private struggles, and the hopes and goals of each family, without imposing our own will upon them. In some circumstances, a family and child are mutually connected with each other, with a shared goal for reunification. In those situations, strategies for enhancing existing strengths and offering new skills are often welcome and utilized. This is enormously gratifying for everyone involved. However, when the vision is not shared between the parent, child, and the department of social services, the challenges can seem unmanageable. We maintain that when a child expresses a desire to connect with their family, regardless of their circumstance, it is our moral responsibility to pursue a safe way to navigate the sometimes treacherous waters. If we were to hold too tightly to our virtuous opinions of how things "should" be before a relationship can be approached, we stand the chance of further distancing the youth from us, and from their pursuits. It is understood that this may cause emotional distress, disruption, anxiety, and unwanted turbulence in the youth's life. However, we hold true to the notion that it is far better for them to attempt to negotiate these complex relationships while we remain in the background, prepared to provide support, rather than driving them to sign themselves out of foster care before they are prepared and leaving them to pursue these often painful connections on their own. For families who are present, and those who are absent, we facilitate progress whenever possible.

Communication is an essential element to successful coparenting. The more effective we are with expressing our thoughts and comprehending the messages our families deliver, the more likely and rapidly we are able to effect meaningful change. This communication is offered through regular telephone contact, home-based family therapy sessions, modeling of successful parenting strategies, and the presentation of a united front to the child in our care. When trust and acceptance are present, and communication flows freely between family and staff, the ingredients exist for successful family empowerment and enduring change.

**The Extra Mile**

By keeping hearts and hands open to our youth, even years after discharge, we provide a home base that serves as a touchstone. Our relationships and strengths-building initiatives do not end when a child leaves our home. For most of our youth an invisible string begins to tug at them late in their adolescence, and their thoughts are filled with the anticipated glory of freedom from the foster care system. For youth without a secure family of permanence, this departure is especially troubling. As their 18th birthday draws near, images of independence that are detached from reason compel so many of our teenagers to sign themselves out of care. Fantasies including living with girlfriends or boyfriends are nearly impossible to compete with as we find ourselves pleading with them to stay until they have the skills they need to survive on their own. Sadly, it's not long after some teens discharge themselves from the system that our phones begin to ring from our libertines whose friends abandoned them, leaving them ill-equipped to live independently. When they reconnect with the group home team, their innate strengths have a chance to become recharged and refocused. Like flowers to the sun, the opportunity to bask in the emotional support of the team strengthens our youth as they move along in their complicated lives.

## Leadership

A strengths-based philosophy is not only a driving force for guiding the children in our care, but also for those of us who lead the organization. As an effective leader I've had to come to terms with my weaknesses, and learn to use my strengths in order to develop my skills, and the capacities of those I supervise. This can be a humbling experience. If we allow it, the helm can be an isolating place. For me it has been the moments of camaraderie among our youth, our caregivers, mentors, and colleagues that have helped me to grow. Our shoulders bear the cumulative load of responsibility that reach far beyond our own actions, extending to the decisions and behaviors of each of our staff. But with a collaborative approach, the weight is distributed and the mutual investment in the organization's success is high. For me that has meant calling on my colleagues for advice, leaning on clinicians for direction, trusting in my board of directors to support me, and communicating openly with all staff and youth. This means face-to-face interactions with children and child care counselors every week. It requires complete transparency with the governing board. It means including all levels of staff within the organization in making decisions about program development. It has also meant embracing the notion that department leaders from different, albeit competing, organizations can and should collaborate to raise the collective bar on the quality of services we provide. One of our most cherished values is to create a home for healing that is also a place of reverence that honors not only the strengths of a child but embraces the unique and special person who walks through our door and sits at our table, including his or her suffering, often borne with dignity and courage.

## Tomorrow

Through my mind's eye I can look into the years ahead to see all of our children flourished into happy adults, each of them finding their own unique path. I see their resilient smiles, and they are able to handle life's mountains and valley's better than most others; wise beyond their years and content at long last. I imagine them free from the binds of growing up within a system of care and restoring the joy of their lost childhoods in children of their own. I hope to find them one day able to forgive us for our inadequacies and our inconsistencies, having learned from our fallibilities that life gives and takes, and that what doesn't bend breaks.

# 18

# The Use of Positive Ethics in the Supervision of Doctoral Psychology Interns

*Athena A. Drewes*

Historically, since the 1950 Boulder Conference, the practice and scope of clinical psychology has come to be characterized by four basic assumptions regarding the nature of psychological adjustment and maladjustment (Barone, Maddux, & Snyder, 1997). First, clinical psychology was concerned with "psychopathology—deviant, abnormal, and maladaptive behavioral and emotional conditions" (Maddux, 2002, p. 14). Second, "psychopathology, clinical problems, and clinical populations differ in kind, not just in degree" (Maddux, 2002, p. 14) from normal populations and problems. Third, "psychological disorders are analogous to biological or medical diseases and reside somewhere *inside* the individual" (Maddux, 2002, p. 14). And fourth, that it is the clinician's task to "identify (diagnose) the disorder (disease) inside the person (patient) and to prescribe an intervention (treatment) that will eliminate (cure) the internal disorder (disease)" (Maddux, 2002, p. 14). It has been hard since then for clinical psychology to move away from these basic assumptions.

Luckily over the past decade there has been a movement toward viewing the client in a more positive light and moving away from focusing on psychological and behavioral deficits. This movement has become a positive psychology whereby the competence of the child and his or her family is focused on along with enhancing growth in psychological domains (Roberts, Brown, Johnson, & Reinke, 2002).

## POSITIVE PSYCHOLOGY

Positive psychology studies the ordinary human strengths and virtues of average people in order to find out "what works, what is right, and what is improving" (Sheldon & King, 2001, p. 216). Positive psychology is an attempt to get psychologists to adopt a more open and appreciative perspective of human potential, motives, and capacities, just as a physicist might admire the elegance of Einstein's equations or an archeologist might marvel at ancient people's accomplishments (Sheldon & King, 2001). It is difficult to see normal functioning of individuals when we focus exclusively on the negative or through a problem-focused lens (Sheldon & King, 2001). Psychologists have for the most part focused most of their attention and energies on the "diagnosis and treatment of pathologies and, in the quest for 'fixes,' scant attention has been paid to the nature of psychological health" (Sheldon & King, 2001, p. 216).

We need to be "looking at strengths rather than deficits, opportunities rather than risks, assets rather than liabilities" (Johnson & Roberts, 1999, p. 5) not only in child psychology, but across the fields of psychotherapy, education, and parenting literature (Roberts et al., 2002). A positive psychology approach allows us as clinicians to focus on the child while he or she is developing and thereby enhancing the child's functioning, competence, and overall mental health at any particular time (Roberts et al., 2002). This more affirming and strengths-building or strengths-based approach should also be conveyed within schools where children can experience empowerment and enhanced development rather than having the emphasis and focus be on stresses and challenges (Roberts et al., 2002; Schorr, 1997; Snyder & Lopez, 2002).

The field of psychology also needs to shift its approach with regard to professional ethics and supervision. The goal needs to be to shift from the current view of an "almost exclusive focus on wrongdoing and disciplinary responses to a more balanced and integrative approach that includes encouraging psychologists to aspire to their highest ethical potential" (Handelsman, Knapp, & Gottlieb, 2002, p. 731).

## ETHICS

Ethics is a general term that refers to values, how we ought to behave, and what is proper conduct. Practical or applied ethics refers to the application of ethics to specialized areas or professions, such as psychology. Psychologists are helped to reach a higher level of service by attending to the practical ethical issues that arise as we deliver health care, teach, conduct research, or engage in other professional activities (Knapp & VandeCreek, 2006). Ethical principles and behavior are hallmarks of professional practices and are frequently discussed in the counseling, social work, and psychology literature (Stewart, 2008). It is also important for psychologists to understand the moral principles on which the standards of the American Psychological Association Ethics Code (2002) are based, and to view it from the standpoint of principle-based ethics (Knapp & VandeCreek, 2006). The APA Ethics Code (2002) addresses ethically complex issues such as competence, multiple relationships, informed consent, confidentiality, fees and financial issues, and public statements (Knapp & VandeCreek, 2006).

## Remedial or Negative Ethics

But psychologists also use the word ethics to refer to both the mandatory or minimum standards adopted by the profession (i.e., remedial ethics), as well as to voluntary efforts to live out moral ideals (Knapp & VandeCreek, 2006). The remedial approach focuses almost exclusively on the laws or standards designed to protect the public from harmful actions by psychologists. That is, doing just enough to avoid any trouble that might come from a violation of ethical standards. Or, doing just the bare minimum to make oneself competent for a particular activity (e.g., taking courses, getting supervision) (Handlesman, Knapp, & Gottlieb, 2002).

Negative ethics, in a sense, has a narrow focus that is limited to codes and laws, enforceable rules and standards. It is focused on misconduct and problems, and the identification of specifically prohibited activities along with sanctions for misconduct. Its goal is to screen out the bad psychologists. There is limited discussion of ethical issues, and it separates out the personal from the professional along with an emphasis on the denial or devaluation of self-interest (Handelsman, Knapp, & Gottlieb, 2002).

However, ethics "can also be viewed as a voluntary effort to 'do the right thing,' motivated by deeply held moral principles" (Knapp & VandeCreek, 2006, p. 3). A positive approach is one whereby the individual makes every effort to assure that one's professional behavior is as consistent with ethical principles as possible. Thus a psychologist with a positive approach to ethics would strive to become as competent as possible (e.g., additional courses, extra supervision, self-study, and self-care). Rather than deliberate on wrongdoings and disciplinary measures and procedures, positive ethics concentrates on respectful relationships and action; that is, doing the right thing.

## Positive Ethics

Positive ethics, in contrast to remedial or negative ethics, has a comprehensive focus, integrating codes with one's personal and cultural ethical traditions. Aspirational principles, virtues, and values are the emphasis, with focus on conduct, positive behaviors, and ethical ideals.

Psychologists are encouraged toward self-care in order to better take care of those they serve. The benefits of ethical reasoning and behavior are encouraged on a personal and professional level. There is broad discussion of ethical issues, focusing on an integration of the awareness of personal and professional ethical principles, while recognizing and integrating appropriate self-interest (such as one's positive motivations for optimal professional behavior) (Handelsman, Knapp, & Gottlieb, 2002). The precursor of positive ethics is positive psychology.

Positive ethics differs from aspirational ethics in that it encourages psychologists to integrate personal ideals into their professional lives. Positive ethics requires a fundamental philosophical underpinning, which can include virtue ethics or any philosophical system. However, it is often a system based on or influenced by personal religious convictions or personal cultural backgrounds and upbringing and altered through personal experiences. These values can become central to the individual's self-concept (Knapp & VandeCreek, 2006). An important feature of positive ethics is that it encourages the individual to integrate their professional ethics with the ethical beliefs that guide their personal lives.

The remedial approach reflects an incomplete view of ethics. Most psychologists want to do more than just avoid being punished. Rather they want to make a positive impact on others and to excel in their profession (Knapp & VandeCreek, 2006). Ethics should be viewed as a way to help psychologists fulfill their highest potential, reach moral excellence, and not just meet the minimal obligations (Knapp & VandeCreek, 2006).

## ETHICAL DILEMMAS

Too often clinicians and students find themselves caught in situations where it appears that in order to comply with a good and valid ethical principle one must violate another principle they also support. At other times, their personal values appear to conflict with the legal or societal requirements of our profession.

Psychologists have to confront and deal with ethical dilemmas each day. A positive approach helps psychologists clarify what they value, consider how they should behave in their role, and determine what constitutes proper professional conduct (Knapp & VandeCreek, 2006). Positive ethics, an innovative ethical perspective, focuses on the affirmative individual traits, such as integrity and courage, in professional actions that enables psychologists to reach their highest ethical ideals, rather than avoid breaking rules (Knapp & VandeCreek, 2006).

The 2002 Ethics Code of the American Psychological Association is the underlying guide to positive ethics as formulated by Knapp and VandeCreek. They lay out a five-step model for resolving ethical dilemmas, illustrating both ethical and questionable behaviors. The importance of self-care, which involves self-regulation, allows for emotional competence and taking time to understand the unique occupational challenges of being a psychologist.

## SUPERVISION

Clinical supervision is the ongoing relationship between a senior member with an apprentice or junior member of the profession, whereby the supervisor mentors and oversees the quality of the treatment given by the apprentice or junior member. In addition, the supervisor's goal is to enhance professional functioning, as well as to ensure the qualifications of the junior member in order to become an independently practicing professional (Knapp & VandeCreek, 2006). The supervisory relationship can have a long-term impact on the life of supervisees. Many supervisees recall encountering difficult patients and determining how to respond to these cases by recalling the words (hearing the voice) of their supervisors. "Supervisors are often the role models for their supervisees and are crucial in forming their professional identity" (Knapp & VandeCreek, 2006, p. 218).

Ethics education should be life-long and provide students and trainees with positive, ongoing, experiential, and supportive educational environments and activities (Gottlieb, Handelsman, & Knapp, 2008). Positive ethics facilitates effective supervision that is personally meaningful, principled, and culturally responsive for both the supervisor and supervisee. Furthermore the knowledge and skills are applicable to both teamwork and selected client interactions (Stewart, 2008). Emphasis is placed on the client and therapist collaborating to identify mutually agreed upon goals and intervention strategies.

Positive ethics requires self-reflection and discernment of personal values. Within supervision the supervisee should be encouraged to create their personal narratives of ethical behavior, reflecting on and relating when they believe they were, indeed, doing the right thing. The supervisor helps ascertain with the intern the influence of cultural values, and ways to help ensure that training and supervision is a positive professional and personal development experience (Stewart, 2008).

Within clinical supervision, the student needs to be encouraged to explore their own motivations and self-perceptions and "to ask basic questions: Why did we go into this profession in the first place? How do we see ourselves as professionals? How do we understand the concept of being helpful?"(Handelsman, Knapp, & Gottlieb, 2002, p. 735). This discussion allows the emerging clinician to put self-interest into perspective, rather than letting financial interests compromise or cloud judgment. The supervisor can help the student to prioritize moral values relative to other values, and help to clarify their moral and ethical values, thereby making them prominent in their thinking which can help align behaviors (Handelsman, Knapp, & Gottlieb, 2002). Rule-based or principle-based ethics invites us to ask the question, what should (or shouldn't) I do? It values clarification and invites us to ask, what do I believe? Along with virtue ethics it takes us to the next step, inviting us to ask, who should I be? "The personal qualities that enable positive ethical behavior include, but are not limited to, humility, prudence, respectfulness, integrity, and benevolence" (Handelsman, Knapp, & Gottlieb, 2002, p. 736). We need to help our supervisees to persevere in the face of distractions, and to implement their skills, while having the courage to act ethically in the face of competing forces (Handelsman, Knapp, & Gottlieb, 2002).

Supervisees and students will make clinical errors and ethical misjudgments. These become "teachable moments," as long as there is an open, supportive, and honest relationship between the supervisor and supervisee. Through the self-disclosure of the supervisor, the supervisee learns to take risks in sharing their mistakes, and trusting their own intuition and judgment in the face of possible personal consequences (Drewes, 2008). The behavior of psychologists as teachers or supervisors should be guided by virtues and ethical principles as should the behavior of psychologists in other venues (Gottlieb, Handelsman, & Knapp, 2008).

A supervisory model follows that addresses how best to achieve this goal.

## ENHANCING SUPERVISEE EXCELLENCE

### Ethics Acculturation Model

The Ethics Acculturation Model (EAM) is based on the premise that psychology "represents a discrete culture with its own traditions, values, and methods of implementing its ethical principles" (Handelsman, Gottlieb, & Knapp, 2005, p. 59).

Ethics training for interns may be more effective if it is designed and "offered from a positive perspective; process-oriented and experiential; supportive; sensitive to the backgrounds and experiences of each student; and understood as a lifelong process (Gottlieb, Handelsman, & Knapp, 2008, p. 123).

John Berry's (1980, 2003) model of cultural adaptation and acculturation, which underlies EAM, proposes that ethics training for students needs to help the student integrate their own ethical and value traditions with those of professional psychology. This model has two major variables that underlie the acculturation model. "The first variable, *maintenance* refers to the degree to which people retain the ethical and value traditions of their culture of origin" (Gottlieb, Handelsman, & Knapp, 2008, p.123). Each student has existing notions of right and wrong professional behavior that is based upon their own personal family values, ethnicity, national origin, religious traditions, and personal role models. The second variable, *contact and participation,* has to do with the degree to which students adopt the traditions, norms, and values of their new professional culture (Gottlieb, Handelsman, & Knapp, 2008; Handelsman, Gottlieb, & Knapp, 2005).

Mitchell Handelsman, Michael Gottlieb, and Samuel Knapp (2005) adapted Berry's model, coming up with four categories or strategies of ethical acculturation. Students high on both maintenance and contact utilize an *integration strategy*. This is the ideal level whereby the student or intern has the highest combination of personal and professional identities. With regard to professional and ethical acculturation, the student can adopt the ethical values of psychology while maintaining much of their own value traditions, thereby coming to a richer and deeper appreciation of the underlying principles of both cultures (Handelsman, Gottlieb, & Knapp, 2005, 2008). For example: Psychologists who follow integration strategies will follow the requirements of documenting consent and providing information to the client, not because they are required by the APA Ethics Code (APA, 2002), their state laws, or any other sources, but because they see following these procedures as the natural extension of their own personal values of advocacy for the client's self-determination. Lower down on the continuum, and less optimal alternatives, are *separation* and *assimilation* (Berry & Sam, 1997; Handelsman, Gottlieb, & Knapp, 2005). The first, *separation,* results in high maintenance and low contact, whereby the student makes professional decisions based primarily on their own personal morals and value traditions, but do not identify as strongly with or incorporate the values of professional psychology. For example, the student may make decisions solely based on their own personal experiences or values, believing their own judgments are sufficient, as it has been in other relationships. Such a viewpoint can lead to becoming uninformed or even feeling disdain toward the ethical and legal constraints put upon them, resulting in a lack of awareness of the potential harm they can cause to their clients (Gottlieb, Handelsman, & Knapp, 2008).

*Assimilation* (Berry & Sam, 1997; Handelsman, Gottlieb, & Knapp, 2005) results in the student over-identifying with professional standards to such an extreme that the student loses much of their own moral identity, and divorces themselves from their personal moral identity feeling that they are no longer necessary (Gottlieb, Handelsman, & Knapp, 2008). Students literally comply while lacking moral foundations which can then lead to an overly simplistic application of professional ethical principles (Handelsman, Gottlieb, & Knapp, 2005; Gottlieb, Handelsman, & Knapp, 2008). As a result students, for example, would conscientiously and rotely obtain informed consent, but would overlook the clinical benefits of encouraging the client to ask questions and involve the client in the decision-making process (Gottlieb, Handelsman, & Knapp, 2008).

The final acculturation strategy is *marginalization*, which can be most problematic for students. This is low identification with both personal and professional cultures, whereby the student has neither a well-developed personal moral sense nor an internalized professional ethic. Thus the student may follow the ethics code "out of personal convenience rather than a sense of moral commitment" (Handelsman, Gottlieb, & Knapp, 2005, p. 61).

Ethics education needs to be experiential. Emotionally charged experiences are crucial components of ethical deliberation (Betan & Stanton, 1999) resulting in the student becoming more fully engaged and effective when they experience the choices they make both intellectually and emotionally. Experiential and positive ethics training may help psychologists develop or hone their integration skills by being more open about their values, motivations, conflicts, and aspirations (Pope, Sonne, & Greene, 2006; Gottlieb, Handelsman, & Knapp, 2008). Such discussions and experiential training, however, needs to be done in a socially supportive environment, which can foster sound ethical decision making, good risk management, and attentive self-care through the experience and expression of positive emotion. Such positive emotion can help build a reservoir of strength and resilience that can be drawn upon in times of stress (Gottlieb, Handelsman, & Knapp, 2008).

## PERSONAL EXAMPLE

At some point during the training year, in my twice-monthly group play therapy supervision of doctoral psychology interns, I self-disclose this personal example to help them begin to think about and articulate their own personal morals and sense of integrity. And to help them aspire to be the best psychologist possible. I stress that at some point in their lives they will need to take a personal stand. They may need to be willing to risk their job as they advocate for the children and clients they serve in order to uphold their personal integrity. This example becomes the basis of deep personal discussions in thinking about positive ethics and the formulation of their own personal ethics as psychologists. It is an experience that I continually draw on, personally, in reaffirming my own personal moral values and beliefs.

I share with them first the basis of my own ethics and morals, my strong underlying personal and religious belief in the inherent worth and dignity of each and every person. And that the respect that I give is not just to the parent or family members, but especially to each child I encounter in my professional and personal life.

A few years after having gotten my master's in clinical psychology, and five years before returning to school for a doctorate (now 22 years ago) I was working in an outpatient clinic in an upstate New York county. I was the designated child play therapist for treatment and assessment, as no one else had those skills. Consequently all young children were given to me. One day a referral came in for me to evaluate a boy of almost five years of age for schizophrenia. The child had been seen in speech therapy by a prominent speech therapist in a local hospital for over two years. She was not having much success with him in speech therapy, noting little progress, and believed him to be schizophrenic and probably autistic. She felt that he was of limited intelligence based on the mother's low intellectual and socioeconomic level. In short, she had already diagnosed him and wanted verification, while at the same time having passed judgment on the parent.

The child came into my office for the designated evaluation. He separated easily from his mother, who was apprehensive about the possibility that I would diagnose him mentally retarded, a stigma she personally had to adversely live with for most of her life. It was evident upon meeting her that her love for her son was paramount, and that while she might have been labeled mentally retarded at some point in her life, she had many strengths and common sense to manage in the world.

As the testing began, the child seemed to be in his own world. He wandered around the room, making comments about the painting on the wall, touching it and even sniffing it, which appeared somewhat bizarre. Testing was slow and tedious as he responded to test questions with non sequitur responses that were strange. However, as I started to tune in more to his responses, I realized that his answers were actually to questions asked much earlier, not to the current one. While the answer seemed initially bizarre, it was actually somewhat relevant to the earlier question. I also began to listen to how he spoke. His tone of voice was rather flat, atonal, without inflection. It gnawed at me. Due to the child's limited ability to respond to the testing material, I pondered whether he was indeed going to score low and considered that maybe he was autistic. If I stopped at this point, between his test results and observations of his behaviors, I could have easily gone with autism, and even childhood schizophrenia. I had many more clients to see with a busy day ahead. How easy it would have been to just take a shortcut and confirm the speech therapist's impressions.

However, I trusted the gnawing feeling within that said to me that this boy was deaf. I had never heard children or adults speak who were marginally hearing or deaf, so I really didn't have a basis to make that assumption.

But I trusted my instincts. I was not going to send this child on the life-altering path of being labeled schizophrenic without a brain-stem audiological examination to definitively rule out hearing loss. The report stated he had normal hearing according to the speech therapist.

I stated to the mother that before my evaluation could be completed, I needed this specialized hearing evaluation conducted at the local hospital. I was adamant that I would not give him a diagnosis without it. The hearing test entails lightly anesthetizing the child, hooking up electrodes to the brain stem, and seeing whether tones and sounds were registering directly at the brain-stem level, for example, being heard. It was a more accurate measure than the traditional hearing tests, with headphones to hear sounds and lights to respond to, that are given to children. The mother went back to the speech therapist and reported my recommendation.

The clinic director called me into her office a few days later. She told me that the referring speech therapist was livid. How dare I challenge her and her professional opinion! Who was I to think he was deaf? She had been working with him for over two years. He could hear. She demanded that I be fired.

I stood my ground, willing to risk my job, and professional career, for my personal integrity, beliefs, and morals. I told the director my reasons that I suspected he was deaf. I was adamant that I was not going to give him a diagnosis that could severely impact the direction of his life into a world of life-long medication and probable institutions without this test first. The director was swayed by my strong personal ethical and moral beliefs in this case, and backed my decision.

The child had the brain-stem hearing evaluation and the results came back. He was profoundly deaf in one ear and moderately deaf in the other.

As you can imagine, the mother was extremely grateful that this was discovered, and that her son would receive the help he needed to make up for lost time for not learning due to this significant deficit (and not because of her own limitations). I breathed a sigh of relief that I hadn't sent this boy on the road of forever being considered schizophrenic. While I felt vindicated in having taken my strong stand, the experience taught me a critical lesson that significantly impacted my professional life. First, to trust and listen to my "gut" instincts, even if it might go against others or previously received information and to hold firm to my personal convictions, morals, and integrity. Next to not assume pathology or blindly accept another's diagnosis. Rather, to rule out physical or medical possibilities first. And finally to hold my ground and fight for what I believe is in the best interest of the client, against all odds, even at personal expense.

A year later the mother contacted me again, as the public school wanted to classify her son as mentally retarded. Again I became the advocate for the child and mother, and went to the Committee on Special Education meeting. I forcibly argued that while the boy was indeed functioning at a lower intellectual level (with his bizarre mannerisms having abated once he got hearing aids), that his significant hearing deficit, and loss of early education, warranted a "multiply handicapped" state classification over a strictly MR classification (which again would push him in another direction educationally). This classification was granted, which allowed a broader range of educational services for him. And it helped the mother avoid the pain of a stigma she had to live with.

## SUMMARY

Ethics education has become too heavily focused on rule adherence in order to help students avoid professional sanctions and civil litigation, which can inadvertently foster and reinforce an assimilation strategy. Ethics can and should be taught from a more positive and aspirational perspective (Gottlieb, Handelsman, & Knapp, 2008).

A positive ethics approach is needed (Handelsman, Knapp, & Gottlieb, 2002) thereby shifting the primary emphasis from avoiding professional discipline to a "more balanced and integrative approach that includes encouraging psychologists to aspire to their highest ethical potential" (Handelsman, Knapp, & Gottlieb, 2002, p. 731; Gottlieb, Handelsman, & Knapp, 2008, p. 124).

By helping students and interns to have positive ethics, it allows for the awareness of the ways that the profession's enforceable rules are based on its higher aspirational principles (Gottlieb, Handelsman, & Knapp, 2008). Positive ethics can allow the student a greater degree of openness so that they and colleagues can be more free to explore difficult issues (e.g., Gottlieb, Handelsman, & Knapp, 2008; Pope, Sonne, & Green, 2006) as well as seek out the assistance of others. And most importantly, it also may help students "consider ethical issues in a broader context, for example, by more explicitly including their highest personal and professional values, virtues, and motivations into their decision making" (Gottlieb, Handelsman, & Knapp, 2008, p. 125).

## REFERENCES

American Psychological Association. (2002). Ethical principles of psychologists and code of conduct. *American Psychologist, 57,* 1060–1073.

Barone, D. F., Maddux, J. E., & Snyder, C. R. (1997). *Social cognitive psychology: History and current domains.* New York: Plenum.

Berry, J. W. (1980). Acculturation as variety of adaptation. In A. M. Padilla (Ed.), *Acculturation: Theory, models, and some new findings* (pp. 9–25). Boulder, CO: Westview Press.

Berry, J. W. (2003). Conceptual approaches to acculturation. In K. M. Chun, P. B. Organista, & G. Marin (Eds.), *Acculturation: Advances in theory, measurement, and applied research* (pp. 291–326). Needham Heights, MA: Allyn & Bacon.

Berry, J. W., & Sam, D. L. (1997). Acculturation and adaptation. In J. W. Berry, M. H. Segall, & C. Kagiticibas (Eds.), *Handbook of cross-cultural psychology* (pp. 291–326). Boston: Allyn & Bacon.

Betan, E. J., & Stanton, A. L. (1999). Fostering ethical willingness: Integrating emotional and contextual awareness of rational analysis. *Professional Psychology: Research & Practice, 20*(5), 283–293.

Drewes, A. A. (2008). Culturally competent supervision of child and play therapists. In A. A. Drewes & J. A. Mullen (Eds.), *Supervision can be playful: Techniques for child and play therapist supervisors* (pp. 77–90). Lanham, MD: Jason Aronson.

Gottlieb, M., Handelsman, M., & Knapp, S. (2008). Some principles for ethics education: Implementing the acculturation model. *Training and Education in Professional Psychology, 2*(3), 123–128.

Handelsman, M. M., Gottlieb, M. C., & Knapp, S. (2005). Training ethical psychologists: An acculturation model. *Professional Psychology: Research and Practice, 36*, 59–65.

Handelsman, M. M., Knapp, S., & Gottlieb, M. C. (2002). Positive ethics. In C. R. Snyder & S. H. Lopez (Eds.), *Handbook of positive psychology* (pp. 731–744). New York: Oxford University Press.

Johnson, N. G., & Roberts, M. C. (1999). Passage on the wild river of adolescence: Arriving safely. In N. G. Johnson, M. C. Roberts, & J. Worrell (Eds.), *Beyond appearances: A new look at adolescent girls* (pp. 3–18). Washington, DC: American Psychological Association.

Knapp, S. J., & VandeCreek, L. D. (2006). *Practical Ethics for Psychologists: A positive approach*. Washington, DC: American Psychological Association.

Maddux, J. E. (2002). Stopping the "madness": Positive psychology and the deconstruction of the illness ideology and the DSM. In C. R. Snyder & S. H. Lopez (Eds.), *Handbook of positive psychology* (pp. 13–25). New York: Oxford University Press.

Pope, K. S., Sonne, J. L., & Greene, B. (2006). *What therapists don't talk about and why*. Washington, DC: American Psychological Association.

Roberts, M. C., Brown, K. J., Johnson, R. J., & Reinke, J. (2002). Positive psychology for children. Development, prevention, and promotion. In C. R. Snyder & S. H. Lopez (Eds.), *Handbook of positive psychology* (pp. 663–686). New York: Oxford University Press.

Schorr, L. B. (1997). *Common purpose: Strengthening families and neighborhoods to rebuild America*. New York: Anchor Books/Doubleday.

Sheldon, K., & King, L. (2001). Why positive psychology is necessary. *American Psychologist, 56*(3), 216–217.

Snyder, C. R., & Lopez, S. H. (2002). *Handbook of positive psychology*. New York: Oxford University Press.

Stewart, A. (2008). Personal communication.

# Epilogue: Reverence for Healers

*David A. Crenshaw*

A book about reverence in healing would not be complete without reverence for the healers. The work of healing the emotional wounds of others requires the full engagement of heart and mind of the healer, and a sensitive attunement to the wounded person as well as the capacity for empathic understanding and responding. The work is emotionally taxing and can be exhausting. Healers are not exempt from the wounds that have stricken those they seek to help. In addition to the work done with the seeker of help; the helper must constantly self-monitor his or her own reactions and responses to sort out what may be interferences with understanding and helping the other that originate within the self. This is a very tall order. Healing can't be done without a considerable emotional toll. Self-care becomes essential. Every therapist should develop a self-care package that would include such items as adequate nutrition, rest, exercise, satisfying relationships with family and friends, fun, supervision and consultation with colleagues, and continuing education.

Milton Erickson, the celebrated hypnotherapist, whose work had a major impact on family therapy and solution-focused therapy, was stricken with polio in his youth. In his writings he described the agonizing process of teaching himself to walk again. It took amazing powers of attention and focus to accomplish this, but he did. These same powers of concentrated focus were called on again by him in later life when he was once again bedridden and his daughter would bring him each morning his favorite flower from his garden, which he used to tend to so lovingly. It was the Night Blooming Cereus, a variety of cactus plant that only blooms at night, but what a show of color and beauty it bestows on its admirers. If you are not familiar with this plant, that is rather homely looking until it blooms, you may want to treat yourself by doing an online search for the Night Blooming Cereus and just enjoy its spectacular beauty.

Erickson reported that he was able to focus with such intensity on this incredible transformation from the plain to the gorgeous beauty, when this flower bloomed in the night, that he was able to experience the same degree of pleasure that he gained from tending his garden when he was still able to walk.

I was always deeply moved by this story. Originally I thought it was a single red rose that his daughter brought Erickson each morning but when I spoke with Dr. Jeffrey Zweig, president of the Erickson Foundation, at the 2009 Psychotherapy Networker Symposium, he told me it was the Night Blooming Cereus. I believe there is much to inspire us about the Erickson story. In our work we have many encounters with the unseemly side of humanity, the dark, sometimes scary, and at times outright ugliness of human beings inflicting cruelty on others. Yet, there is beauty all around us. Like the single Night Blooming Cereus there is beauty galore to be absorbed, attended to, concentrated on, and too precious to overlook. Beauty beckons us all in countless ways, sometimes coming in transformations like the Night Blooming Cereus that is a wonder to behold, beauty in the world, beauty in people, beauty within us too important to ignore.

For just a moment, please turn a kind gaze inward and notice the inward beauty of a person who has dedicated your professional life to helping others. It takes a special person to do what you do; this is a calling, not a job, and the majority of people would not be able to heed the call, but you did. Appreciate the kind and giving heart that resides within you. You may never know the difference you make in the life of a child or adult. There are children and adults who years later still hear inside them the voice of their therapist and certain words that were particularly meaningful to them. Many more will not remember your words but they will never forget how much you cared. Notice your colleagues who have cast their lot along side of you. Men and women, just like you, so generous and giving of heart. Appreciate the beauty within and around you because it is precious. Each of you arises in the morning and goes to work with the knowledge that today you may make a difference in the life of child or a family. May you be blessed for all that you give and the good work you do. May the incredible beauty of the Night Blooming Cereus symbolize for you the beauty within.

# Index

# About the Contributors

**Megan Barbera**, LCSW, has an extensive background in child and family preventive mental health care and has authored and presented research conducted in these areas to help guide the formation of several ongoing county-administered early intervention/prevention programs in Northern Colorado. Currently, she is in private practice in Rhinebeck, New York, where she specializes in women's issues, with a research focus on mind-body connection, stress reduction, creativity, and relational empowerment during young and middle adulthood. She holds dual clinical licensure in New York and Colorado.

**Gregory Barker**, Ph.D., received his doctorate in school/clinical child psychology from the University of Virginia in 1981. For over 25 years he has specialized in working with children and adolescents in residential, hospital, college counseling, and school settings. For 17 years Dr. Barker consulted to the Bard College Counseling Center and is currently a school psychologist in the Rondout Valley public schools. He also has a private practice in Rhinebeck, New York, where he specializes in working with families and children.

**Robert Brooks**, Ph.D., has lectured nationally and internationally to tens of thousands of parents, educators, and mental health and business professionals on topics pertaining to motivation, resilience, self-worth, family relationships, and balancing our personal and professional lives. He is a member of the faculty of Harvard Medical School and has served as director of the Department of Psychology at McLean Hospital. He is listed in the Council for the National Register of Health Service Providers in Psychology and holds diplomate status in clinical psychology. He has a part-time private practice in which he sees children, adolescents, adults, and females. He has appeared regularly on television in the Boston area as well as on national cable television, and recently completed a videotape and educational guide for the Public Broadcasting Corporation focusing on developing self-worth, hope, and resilience in children with special needs.

**David A. Crenshaw**, Ph.D., ABPP, RPT-S, is director and founder of the Rhinebeck Child and Family Center, LLC, a private practice serving children and families, but also providing training and consultation to agencies serving at-risk children. He is past president of the New York Association for Play Therapy. He is coauthor with John B. Mordock of *A Handbook of Play Therapy with Aggressive Children*, and also *Understanding and Treating the Aggression of Children: Fawns in Gorilla Suits*. He is the author of *Bereavement: Counseling the Grieving throughout the Life Cycle*; *Evocative Strategies in Child and Adolescent Psychotherapy*; and *Therapeutic Engagement of Children and Adolescents: Play, Symbol, Drawing and Storytelling Strategies*; and editor of *Child and Adolescent Psychotherapy: Wounded Spirits and Healing Paths*. He served as clinical director for over 30 years in residential treatment of emotionally disturbed, often abused and traumatized children.

**Susan Cristantiello**, ATR, LCAT, is an art psychotherapist and serves as the CCSI Coordinator for Astor Home Based Services in Dutchess County, New York. She has been in private practice for over 25 years, and has been a professor of art therapy at the College of New Rochelle and Westchester Community College. She was one of the founding members of the Westchester Art Therapy Association, where she served as president, vice president, and program chair of the chapter. She has contributed to the *American Art Therapy Journal*, lectured widely, and has worked as a lecturer, consultant, and training supervisor throughout her career.

**Athena A. Drewes**, Psy.D., is a licensed child psychologist and registered play therapist and supervisor. She is director of clinical training and APA-Accredited Doctoral Internship at Astor Services for Children and Families, a large multiservice nonprofit mental health agency in New York. She has over 25 years clinical experience in working with sexually abused and traumatized children and adolescents in school, outpatient, and inpatient settings. She has been a clinical supervisor for over 15 years. She is a former board of director of the Association for Play Therapy and founder/past president of New York Association for Play Therapy. She has written and lectured extensively in the United States and abroad on play therapy. Her books include *School-Based Play Therapy*; *Cultural Issues in Play Therapy*; *Supervision Can Be Playful: Techniques for Child and Play Therapy Supervisors*;

*Blending Play Therapy with Cognitive Behavioral Therapy: Evidence-Based and Other Effective Treatments and Techniques*; and *School-Based Play Therapy, Second Edition*.

**Renee Fillette**, M.A., is the founder and executive director of St. John Bosco Child and Family Services, an organization whose mission is to provide community-based homes and services to children who have been removed from their families. With her team she has implemented a unique, strengths-based approach to residential child care. Previously she consulted throughout the northeastern United States, Canada, and Iceland in the treatment of young children with autism.

**Andrew Fussner**, MSW, has worked 30 years as a family therapist; 20 years at the Philadelphia Child Guidance Clinic. He currently works as mental health consultant to the Pre-K–kindergarten Head Start program of the School District of Philadelphia, adjunct faculty at the Graduate School of Social Policy and Practice of the University of Pennsylvania, and consultant in family therapy at the Astor Home for Children in Rhinebeck, New York.

**James Garbarino**, Ph.D., holds the Maude C. Clark Chair in Humanistic Psychology and is director of the Center for the Human Rights of Children at Loyola University in Chicago. Previously he was Elizabeth Lee Vincent Professor of Human Development and codirector of the Family Life Development Center at Cornell University. He has authored or edited over 20 books and they include: *See Jane Hit: Why Girls Are Growing More Violent and What We Can Do about It* (2006); *Lost Boys: Why Our Sons Turn Violent and How We Can Save Them* (1999); *Raising Children in a Socially Toxic Environment* (1995); and *Children and the Dark Side of Human Experience* (2008).

**Sueann G. Kenney-Noziska**, MSW, LISW, RPT-S, specializes in using play therapy with abused and traumatized children, adolescents, and families and has over 15 years of experience in the field. She is an accomplished author, instructor of play therapy, guest lecturer, and internationally recognized speaker. Sueann is actively involved in the play therapy community and has held several leadership positions at the state and national levels. She is author of *Techniques-Techniques-Techniques: Play-Based Activities for Children, Adolescents & Families*, a manual which highlights her original techniques and interventions. Sueann is the director and founder of Play Therapy Corner, Inc., in La Mesa, New Mexico.

**Andrew Kuntz**, MCAT, LCSW, holds a master's degree in creative arts therapy and social work, and a post–master's certificate in advanced clinical social work from New York University. In his 30 year career he has directed innovative outpatient programs for children and youth; the past 20 years for the Astor Services for Children and Families. He is currently in charge of the several urban children's outpatient clinic services for the agency in the Bronx, New York.

**Edith C. Lawrence**, Ph.D., is a professor at the University of Virginia's Curry Programs in Clinical and School Psychology and director of the Young Women Leaders Program, a mentoring initiative that pairs middle school girls with college women. She coauthored *Competence, Courage, and Change: An Approach to Family Therapy* (1993) with David Waters and developed the Family Inventory of Resources and Stressors (FIRST), a collaborative, competence-based approach to family assessment.

**Jennifer Lee**, Ph.D., a graduate of Columbia University, is a clinical psychologist in private practice specializing in the treatment of adolescents and families. She also serves as adjunct instructor at Marist College in Poughkeepsie, New York, where she teaches graduate students in mental health counseling. Her research focuses on mindfulness-based interventions, ethnic minority identity development, and adolescent mental health. She has published scientific articles and book chapters on these topics.

**John W. Seymour**, Ph.D., LMFT, is an associate professor in counseling at Minnesota State University, Mankato. He has been a play therapist for over 30 years, and is a registered play therapist-supervisor with the Association for Play Therapy and an approved supervisor with the American Association of Marriage and Family Therapists. Prior to teaching graduate family therapy and play therapy courses at the university, he worked in a variety of settings, including hospital, agency, and residential treatment.

**Misty Solt**, Ph.D., is a licensed professional counselor-supervisor in the state of Texas. Dr. Solt is also a nationally certified counselor and a registered play therapy supervisor. For over a decade, Dr. Solt has worked as a counselor in the following areas: school crisis counseling, in-home counseling, agency counseling, and private practice. Dr. Solt was the assistant director of the Center for Play Therapy for three years and has been a supervisor for the Intensive Play Therapy Supervision component of the Summer Institute for eight years. In May of 2003, Dr. Solt opened the Child and Family Counseling Center in Frisco, Texas, which provides counseling services to children, adolescents, and families, as well as supervision to LPC-interns. Dr. Solt has served on the Frisco Independent School District Hope Rising Team, which is a trauma response team to assist children and teens that have experienced a trauma or loss. Dr. Solt is also on the board of directors for Camp C.O.P.E., which is an intensive counseling experience offered to children of a deployed or injured parent serving in the War in Iraq. Dr. Solt is currently on staff at Southern Methodist University in Plano, Texas, where she serves as the clinic director of the Child and Family Counseling Center and as a lecturer. Dr. Solt has authored various articles in the area of play therapy and is the author of *My Special Playtime*. Dr. Solt is a mother of two and resides in Frisco, Texas.

**John Soracco**, M.A., is currently program director for the Non-Secure Detention program at Astor Services for Children and Families. His background encompasses over 40 years of varied experience including many years of service in the corrections field, as well as working with victims of traumatic brain injury. He holds a B.A. in psychology and an M.A. in education, with certifications as a teacher of the handicapped and a learning disability teacher consultant.

**Amanda F. Sovik-Johnston**, M.Ed., is a graduate student at the University of Virginia in the Curry Programs in Clinical and School Psychology. Her clinical training has included supervising facilitators and mentoring groups for the Young Women Leaders Program. Prior to graduate school she spent seven summers working with children considered emotionally disturbed at Wediko Children's Services Summer Program, a short-term residential treatment center. She also taught special education in the Baltimore City Public School System as well as in the Boston Public Schools.

**E. Mark Stern**, Ed.D., is professor emeritus of the Graduate Faculty of Arts and Sciences, Iona College, New Rochelle. He is a fellow of the American Psychological Association, fellow of the Association for Psychological Science, and a diplomate in clinical psychology of the American Board of Professional Psychology. He was a visiting professor of counseling and psychology at the Catholic University of Australia (Stratford Campus) and has been adjunct professor at Seton Hall and Fordham Universities. Dr. Stern was a founding editor of *The Journal of Pastoral Counseling*, published by Iona College; served for 12 years as editor of *VOICES: The Art and Science of Psychotherapy, the Journal of the American Academy of Psychotherapists*. Subsequently he was founding editor and editor for an additional 12 years of the Psychotherapy Patient Monograph Series, published by the Haworth Press. Dr. Stern has been the president of two divisions of the American Psychological Association, The Division of the Psychology of Religion and the Society for Humanistic Psychology. He has served four terms on the APA Council of Representatives. He has written and published extensively and is the recipient of the Carl Rogers Award and the Virginia Sexton Mentoring Award.

**Lenore Strocchia-Rivera**, Ph.D., has been a licensed psychologist for more than 20 years, the past 11 years as clinical director of the Astor Early Childhood Programs in Dutchess County, New York. Currently she works for the Astor Family Court Evaluation Service. She is also the founder and director of Learning Insights, an evaluation and assessment practice based in Highland, New York, where she specializes in Therapeutic Assessments. Dr. Strocchia-Rivera's experience comes from a wide variety of work settings that include family court, schools, day treatment programs, Head Start, private practice, residential treatment centers, hospitals, and emergency foster care programs. Dr. Strocchia-Rivera has served as adjunct faculty at Marist College, the University of Texas at Austin, and as an advisor-consultant for Empire State College.

**Nancy Tsoubris**, LCSW-R, has been working with children and families for 14 years, beginning her training with the preschool population and specializing in treating families with children and adolescents with severe behavior issues. She is currently in private practice in Rhinebeck, New York, where her work with women, emphasizing the healing power of connection, has become a passion. She is a wife and mother of three young children.

**Steven Tuber**, Ph.D., ABPP, is professor of psychology and past director of the Doctoral Program in Clinical Psychology of the City University of New York at City College. He is the author of *Attachment, Play & Authenticity: A Winnicott Primer* (2008) and has published or presented over 100 papers on the intertwining of diagnosis and treatment in children, adolescents, and adults.

**Donna Zulch**, LCSW-R, has a forensic and clinical social work practice spanning 25 years, with a specialization in the evaluation and treatment of child sexual abuse. She is a former consultant-trainer at Fordham University's Graduate School of Social Services, Center for Training and Research in Child Abuse and Family Violence, and has previously been on the faculty of The State University of New York, Dutchess Community College, serving in the Behavioral Sciences Department and The Center for Business and Industry. She has lectured widely to diverse audiences of legal, judicial, mental health, medical, and educational professionals, and has served as an advisor-consultant for Empire State College and trainer for New York State Department of Education.